Therapeutic Farriery

Guest Editors

STEPHEN E. O'GRADY, DVM, MRCVS, APF
ANDREW H. PARKS, VetMB, MS, MRCVS

VETERINARY CLINICS OF NORTH AMERICA: EQUINE PRACTICE

www.vetequine.theclinics.com

Consulting Editor
ANTHONY SIMON TURNER, BVSc, MS

August 2012 • Volume 28 • Number 2

SAUNDERS an imprint of ELSEVIER, Inc.

W.B. SAUNDERS COMPANY

A Division of Elsevier Inc.

1600 John F. Kennedy Boulevard ● Suite 1800 ● Philadelphia, Pennsylvania 19103

http://www.vetequine.theclinics.com

VETERINARY CLINICS OF NORTH AMERICA: EQUINE PRACTICE Volume 28, Number 2
August 2012 ISSN 0749-0739, ISBN-13: 978-1-4557-3950-9

Editor: John Vassallo; j.vassallo@elsevier.com

Veterinary Clinics of North America: Equine Practice (ISSN 0749-0739) is published in April, August, and December by Elsevier Inc., 360 Park Avenue South, New York, NY 10010-1710. Business and Editorial Offices: 1600 John F. Kennedy Blvd., Suite 1800, Philadelphia, PA 19103-2899. Subscription prices are $267.00 per year (domestic individuals), $397.00 per year (domestic institutions), $126.00 per year (domestic students/residents), $299.00 per year (Canadian individuals), $496.00 per year (Canadian institutions), $346.00 per year (international individuals), $496.00 per year (international institutions), and $172.00 per year (international and Canadian students/residents). To receive student/resident rate, orders must be accompanied by name of affiliated institution, date of term, and the signature of program/residency coordinator on institution letterhead. Orders will be billed at individual rate until proof of status is received. Foreign air speed delivery is included in all *Clinics* subscription prices. All prices are subject to change without notice. **POSTMASTER:** Send address changes to *Veterinary Clinics of North America: Equine Practice*, 3251 Riverport Lane, Maryland Heights, MO 63043. Customer Service (orders, claims, online, change of address): Elsevier Health Sciences Division, Subscription Customer Service, 3251 Riverport Lane, Maryland Heights, MO 63043. Tel: 1-800-654-2452 (U.S. and Canada); 314-447-8871 (outside U.S. and Canada). Fax: 314-447-8029. E-mail: journalscustomer service-usa@elsevier.com (for print support); E-mail: journalsonlinesupport-usa@elsevier (for online support).

Reprints. For copies of 100 or more of articles in this publication, please contact the Commercial Reprints Department, Elsevier Inc., 360 Park Avenue South, New York, NY 10010-1710. Tel.: 212-633-3812; Fax: 212-462-1935; E-mail: reprints@elsevier.com.

Veterinary Clinics of North America: Equine Practice is covered in *MEDLINE/PubMed (Index Medicus)*, *Excerpta Medica, Current Contents/Agriculture, Biology and Environmental Sciences*, and *ISI*.

Printed and bound by CPI Group (UK) Ltd, Croydon, CR0 4YY

Transferred to Digital Print 2012

Contributors

CONSULTING EDITOR

ANTHONY SIMON TURNER, BVSc, MS
Diplomate, American College of Veterinary Surgeons; Professor, Department of Clinical Sciences, College of Veterinary Medicine and Biomedical Sciences, Colorado State University, Fort Collins, Colorado

GUEST EDITORS

STEPHEN E. O'GRADY, DVM, MRCVS, APF
Northern Virginia Equine, Marshall, Virginia

ANDREW H. PARKS, VetMB, MS, MRCVS
Professor, Department of Large Animal Medicine, College of Veterinary Medicine, University of Georgia, Athens, Georgia

AUTHORS

WILLIAM R. BAKER Jr, DVM
Equine Associates LLC, Hawkinsville, Georgia

HANS H. CASTELIJNS, DVM, CF
Equine Podiatry Consult and Referrals, Cortona, Arezzo, Italy

VERNON C. DRYDEN, DVM, CJF
Rood & Riddle Equine Hospital, Lexington, Kentucky

RANDY B. EGGLESTON, DVM
Diplomate, American College of Veterinary Surgeons; Clinical Associate Professor of Large Animal Surgery, Department of Large Animal Medicine, College of Veterinary Medicine, University of Georgia, Athens, Georgia

EHUD ELIASHAR, BSc, DVM, MRCVS
Diplomate of the European College of Veterinary Surgeons; St Albans, Hertfordshire, United Kingdom

ROBERT J. HUNT, DVM, MS
Diplomate, American College of Veterinary Surgeons; Hagyard Equine Medical Institute, Lexington, Kentucky

IAN MCKINLAY
Farrier, South Amboy, New Jersey

WILLIAM A. MOYER, DVM
Diplomate, American College of Veterinary Sports Medicine and Rehabilitation; Professor, Large Animal Clinical Sciences, College of Veterinary Medicine and Biomedical Sciences, Texas A&M University, College Station, Texas

STEPHEN E. O'GRADY, DVM, MRCVS, APF
Northern Virginia Equine, Marshall, Virginia

ANDREW H. PARKS, VetMB, MS, MRCVS
Professor, Department of Large Animal Medicine, College of Veterinary Medicine,
University of Georgia, Athens, Georgia

R. SCOTT PLEASANT, DVM, MS
Diplomate, American College of Veterinary Surgeons; Associate Professor, Department
of Large Animal Clinical Sciences, Virginia-Maryland Regional College of Veterinary
Medicine, Blacksburg, Virginia

HARRY W. WERNER, VMD
Werner Equine LLC, North Granby, Connecticut

W. RICH REDDING, DVM, MS
Diplomate, American College of Veterinary Surgeons; Associate Professor, Department
of Clinical Sciences, College of Veterinary Medicine, North Carolina State University,
Raleigh, North Carolina

Contents

> For an equine practice to offer therapeutic farriery as a professional service, that service must be founded in individual competence and cooperation between veterinarian and farrier. Inadequate farriery education and experience may result in substandard or even contraindicated therapeutic farriery prescriptions and farrier care. Within continuing education for equine practitioners, excellent opportunities to advance one's understanding of and clinical competence in therapeutic farriery are increasingly available. It is the obligation of the veterinarian to acquire and maintain a working understanding of both basic and therapeutic farriery to work effectively with the farrier and offer a valid service to the client.

> Shoes were originally applied to horses' feet to protect against excessive wear. Over the years, countless types of shoes and farriery techniques have been developed not only as a therapeutic aid to treat lameness but also to maintain or enhance functionality. The past 3 decades have provided equine veterinarians and farriers with new information relating to limb biomechanics and the effects of various farriery methods. This article describes the principles of foot biomechanics and how they are affected by some of the more common farriery and shoeing techniques.

> Radiographic evaluation of a horse's foot gives tremendous insight into the relationship between the structures within the foot and between the foot and distal limb. The information gained from a radiographic study is highly dependent on the quality of the radiographs. A systematic approach should be taken when planning a radiographic study of the foot. Taking the time to examine the foot and prepare it properly will avoid the need, risk, and expense of repeating images and will improve the quality and therefore the interpretation of your radiographic images. When evaluating the foot for podiatry reasons, it is crucial that the positioning of the patient, foot, and x-ray beam be flawless.

Domesticated horses need hoof care, because it is rare for wear and growth of the hooves to be in perfect equilibrium. During the shoeing interval, the hoof grows downwards and forward in the direction of the horn tubules, losing some degree of angle. Few horses have perfect limb conformation. The shape of a hoof of a limb with conformation defects adapts in a predictable way. If, for therapeutic or performance reasons, the hoof-shoe combination is modified, there is a not a lot of leeway in the trim of a particular foot, whereas the applied shoe type, placement, and adjustments provide endless possibilities.

Therapeutic shoeing is best directed at a specific diagnosis, but in the absence of a specific diagnosis, it is frequently directed at a symptom. There are only so many ways to modify the function of the foot with trimming and shoeing. The design of a horse shoe may often be modified to improve one aspect of foot function. Modifying a horse shoe to improve one aspect of foot function almost invariably impacts another aspect of foot function. The application of horse shoes may be based on a specific diagnosis or directed at a symptom. The application of shoeing principles is best approached using theoretical reasoning based on the research data that are available and experience.

Underrun heels are common and involve hoof capsule distortion in which the horn tubules of the heels undergo bending and lengthening, resulting in decreased strength and functionality. The syndrome varies in clinical presentation, depending on duration, severity of distortion, presence of secondary problems, and presence of lameness. Primary treatment goals are to maintain soundness and functional integrity of the foot and to establish a normal hoof capsule. Resolution of the problem is generally not achieved in horses in a heavy work schedule, and realistic goals in this situation are to maintain function, alleviate lameness, and arrest progression of the distortion.

A club foot or flexural deformity may affect a horse at any stage of life from neonate through adulthood. The emphasis of this article is on defining and recommending the appropriate farriery for flexural deformities involving the deep digital flexor tendon and the distal interphalangeal joint. Clinical management of the flexural deformity is influenced by the severity, duration, and etiology of the club foot as well as the degree and source of lameness. Also discussed is the management of mismatched hoof angles, which remains a controversial subject for both farrier and veterinarian.

William R. Baker Jr

> Laminitis is typically classified into developmental or prodromal, acute, subacute, and chronic phases. Scientific evidence regarding the patho-physiology of laminitis does exist, but it is often conflicting and dependent on the clinician's interpretation/understanding of the study or the model used for inducing laminitis. The diagnosis of laminitis consists of obtaining an accurate history, performing a thorough physical examination, and taking good-quality radiographs. The use of radiographs for diagnosis and interpretation of laminitis is an absolute necessity for the clinician. Laminitis is one disease that requires the assembly of a team consisting of the veterinarian, the farrier, and the owner to be successfully treated.

VETERINARY CLINICS OF
NORTH AMERICA: EQUINE PRACTICE

THE CLINICS ARE NOW AVAILABLE ONLINE!
Access your subscription at:
www.theclinics.com

Foreword

Therapeutic Farriery

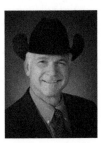

William A. Moyer, DVM

Foot problems represent one of the most common dilemmas that horse owners and trainers encounter and thus seek assistance and expertise from equine practitioners and farriers. Foot problems vary from being "owner" obvious (central toe crack) to situations that are difficult to accurately diagnose even with the latest and greatest imaging technologies. Very few equine practitioners shoe horses and farriers are not legally permitted to provide a diagnosis and treatment beyond trimming and shoeing. Thus the health and welfare of the horse is dependent on a cooperative effort and mutual understanding of specific roles (veterinarian and farrier). The management of many foot problems is or can be difficult and quite challenging.

In the last two decades, we have experienced the introduction of significant advances in imaging modalities that allow enhanced visualization of tissues within the hoof capsule. High-speed and universally available information, as well as a proliferation of products such as improved shoe designs, pads/packing, various types of boots, so-called "natural trimming and shoeing," composites, adhesives, and different means of securing a device to the bottom of the horse's foot, have all become commonplace. Thus the array of available management tools has expanded; unfortunately, most of what we think we know about such products is directly related to marketing rather than science. It is safe to state that veterinary medical education is on curricular overload, accounting for either an absence or a reasonably meager student experience with regard to the basics of trimming and shoeing.

This text is an excellent "state-of-the-art" resource as it is compiled by individuals with extensive experience, honed observational skills, a sincere interest in moving past the anecdotal to the more scientific approach, and, most importantly, a passion for the subject. The range of farriery topics is extensive and varies from how such partners in

Vet Clin Equine 28 (2012) xi–xii
http://dx.doi.org/10.1016/j.cveq.2012.06.009
0749-0739/12/$ – see front matter © 2012 Published by Elsevier Inc.

hoof health can mesh to the involved mechanics of the foot, diagnostic imaging, and a myriad of diseases/injuries that are encountered in an active equine practice.

William A. Moyer, DVM, DACVSMR
College of Veterinary Medicine and Biomedical Sciences
Texas A&M University
College Station, TX, USA

E-mail address:
WMOYER@cvm.tamu.edu

Preface

Therapeutic Farriery

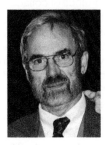 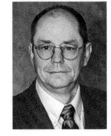

Stephen E. O'Grady, DVM,   Andrew H. Parks, VetMB,
MRCVS, APF   MS, MRCVS

Guest Editors

As a young veterinarian, I (Parks) was advised to pursue an area of interest in which problems are common, in which the problems were important, and that was not glamorous. Diseases of the horse's foot are relatively unglamorous, at least compared with the inviting subjects of the day such as colic surgery and arthroscopy. At that time, an interest in the horse's foot definitely fit all these criteria, although the gradual development of my interest in horse's feet was nowhere near that deliberate. The field has been very rewarding professionally, initially, because it was an area to explore that not many people were interested in and because there were real opportunities to benefit my patients. Latterly, the structure and function of the foot have become intrinsically interesting in their own right—it is simply amazing that a horse can run at 40 miles an hour and land on a single hoof with a diameter of only 4.5 inches with a force of approximately twice its body weight and it doesn't fall apart.

The holy grail of any clinical discipline is to develop systematic approaches to problems, approaches that are instigated by clinical observations and validated by scientific study. It would be optimal if such approaches were linear in development. However, the reality is that they progress in fits and starts, incorporating clinical experience and scientific knowledge as they become available. Fortunately, there have been significant advances in our understanding of foot function over the last 20 years, thanks to several groups of researchers around the world. Additionally, the number of techniques and appliances available to veterinarians and farriers has also proliferated. Furthermore, in the last 10 years or so, interest in the equine foot has also been propelled forward by dramatic advances in equine diagnostic imaging.

The equine foot is composed of many tissues, including bones, joints, ligaments, and tendons, and veterinarians are accomplished at examining and treating these structures elsewhere on the body. So it is the hoof that makes the foot different, in part because it makes all those other structures enclosed within the hoof harder to examine and treat, and in part because of its unique structure, function, and growth. The focus of this issue is to meld clinical knowledge of experienced practitioners and research information

Vet Clin Equine 28 (2012) xiii–xiv
http://dx.doi.org/10.1016/j.cveq.2012.06.008
0749-0739/12/$ – see front matter © 2012 Elsevier Inc. All rights reserved.

available to provide largely practical information about the horse's hoof. Strict adherence to the anatomical structures and the use of biomechanical principles to evaluate the equine foot and apply the appropriate farriery are stressed throughout this issue.

Dr Werner's article provides an excellent introduction to the role of veterinarian and farrier in treating diseases of the equine foot and stresses the importance of collaboration. This is followed by an article by Dr Eliashar that discusses the scientific knowledge for understanding the biomechanical function of the equine foot, knowledge that can be utilized for rational decisions in both basic and therapeutic farriery. The next two articles by Drs Castelijns and Parks describe approaches that they employ for forming goals for basic and therapeutic farriery, respectively; their emphasis is on what you want to achieve rather than how you achieve it. Next, Dr Eggleston writes extensively about the use of imaging and how it is a framework for applying therapeutic farriery.

There are three articles by Drs Hunt, O'Grady, and Dryden on three commonly identified hoof capsule distortions: under-run heels, club feet, and sheared heels; these articles discuss the current thoughts on causes and treatment of these distortions. Dr Pleasant discusses the development and treatment of hoof cracks; hoof cracks are a natural sequel to distortions of the hoof capsule because such distortions are frequently the prelude to a fracture in the hoof wall. Dr Redding has two articles in which he discusses nonseptic and septic diseases of the hoof. Last, Dr Baker tackles laminitis from the perspective of an equine practitioner with substantial experience in treating the disease, including his pragmatic way for managing horses with laminitis.

The guest editors thank Dr Simon Turner for the invitation to edit this issue of the *Veterinary Clinics of North America: Equine Practice*. We would also like to acknowledge the enormous support and contributions of John Vassallo from Elsevier, without whose assistance this volume would never have been completed.

Finally, I (O'Grady) would like to acknowledge two people who have had a huge impact on my life. My coeditor, Dr Andy Parks, who is not only a trusted colleague but a valued friend, has taught me more than I ever imagined about the equine foot. He teaches one to think; he teaches one to ask why, and he continually endeavors to make you the best you can be. And my daughter, Jendaya Regina O'Grady, who gave me the life experience of watching her grow up to be a beautiful mature young lady. She is truly a gift from God.

And I (Parks) for my part would like to thank Dr Steve O'Grady for the countless hours of discussion, thought-provoking questions, and instruction in practical podiatry techniques that may elude those of us in an ivory-tower environment. I also extend my gratitude to my family for their patience and support.

Stephen E. O'Grady, DVM, MRCVS, APF
Northern Virginia Equine
PO Box 746
Marshall, VA 20116, USA

Andrew H. Parks, VetMB, MS, MRCVS
Department of Large Animal Medicine
College of Veterinary Medicine
University of Georgia
501 DW Brooks Drive
Athens, GA 30602-7385, USA

E-mail addresses:
sogrady@look.net (S.E. O'Grady)
parksa@uga.edu (A.H. Parks)

The Importance of Therapeutic Farriery in Equine Practice

Harry W. Werner, VMD

KEYWORDS

- Equine • Farriery • Therapeutic farriery • Continuing education

KEY POINTS

- For an equine practice to legitimately offer therapeutic farriery as a professional service, that service must be founded in individual competence and cooperation between veterinarian and farrier.
- Inadequate farriery education and experience may result in substandard or even contraindicated therapeutic farriery prescriptions and farrier care.
- Within the venue of continuing education for equine practitioners, excellent opportunities to advance one's understanding of and clinical competence in therapeutic farriery are increasingly available.
- It is the obligation of the veterinarian to acquire and maintain a working understanding of the elements of both basic and therapeutic farriery if he or she is to work effectively with the farrier and offer a valid service to the client for their horse.
- For the veterinarian, there should be no tolerance for anything less than the most accurate diagnosis that can be achieved under the circumstances.

INTRODUCTION

The author seeks to define what is meant by therapeutic farriery and to describe how it can—and why it should be —successfully incorporated as a mainstay in equine practice. The intent is not to convert equine practitioners into farriers; rather, the goal is to encourage these two professions to recognize the very real enhancement in equine health care that results when veterinarians and farriers recognize their own and each other's common and unique strengths and work constructively together to deliver the best possible level of therapy.

A brief history of both professions is presented and the current status of veterinary education in therapeutic farriery is discussed. A strong veterinarian–farrier partnership is the foundation on which therapeutic farriery is offered as a professional service; the elements of this partnership—including potential conflicts and resolution—are presented. The importance of acquiring and maintaining competence in

The author has nothing to disclose.
Werner Equine LLC, 20 Godard Road, Box 5, North Granby, CT 06060, USA
E-mail address: hwwvmd@wernerequine.com

Vet Clin Equine 28 (2012) 263–281
http://dx.doi.org/10.1016/j.cveq.2012.05.005
0749-0739/12/$ – see front matter © 2012 Elsevier Inc. All rights reserved.

the biomechanics of the equine digit as well as the current selection of available farriery appliances and materials is stressed. A discussion of the client's expectations, realistic and otherwise, follows and leads into information regarding communications and medical records. Finally, the importance of distinguishing between evidence-based and anecdotal information is emphasized.

HISTORY

Horses are known to have served mankind for millennia. Recent evidence suggests that their domestication was under way as long as 6000 years ago in what is now Ukraine.[1] As their service increased in value, it is reasonable to assume that so, too, did their masters' sense of stewardship. Exactly when human behavior toward the horse evolved to the point where rudimentary attention to the beasts' health and comfort was a cognitive act no doubt predates the written record. However, at some point, human communities began to recognize individuals who demonstrated interest in and some apparent success in working with and maintaining the general well-being of the horse.

Roman military chronicles of the 2nd century AD refer to a place for injured and sick horses, complete with a forge, as a *veterinarium* (**Fig. 1**).[2] A name for such a caregiver first appears in the Middle Ages as *ferrier*, the word deriving from the Anglo-French term for a blacksmith and much earlier from the Latin *ferrum* ("iron"). During the 16th century, the English version became what we know today as a *farrier*.[3] However, long before then and up through the 18th century, society recognized a farrier as someone responsible for the overall health care of the horse—not just the animal's hooves. Even the legal profession saw it that way, as manifest in a lawsuit filed in 1441 during the reign of Henry VI. And in his 1881 text *The Common Law*, Justice Oliver Wendell Holmes refers to it as "the Marshall case," wherein a farrier was sued for negligence and carelessness in treating a horse.[4]

Seventeenth-century England recognized a military person whose duties included attending to both the feet and overall health of the horse. It is clear that the veterinary surgeon of this period was both shoeing-smith and surgeon. Hexam (1637) describes the duties of the Army Farrier as "to drench and lett bloude the horse of the troupe, and alwaies, either upon a march or in quarter, to have in readiness his buggett of tools, horseshoes and nailes, whensoever he shall be called upon by his officers, or when any gentleman of the troupe shall have use of him, and for this reason that he must duly attend upon the Troupe he is freed from other duties and hath a greater paye than an ordinary horseman."[5]

Roman 100 AD

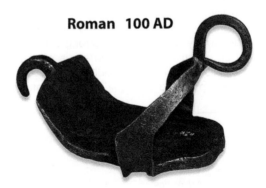

Fig. 1. Roman shoe ca 100 AD.

Formal recognition of an equine health care provider as separate from a farrier occurred in 1761, when the world's first veterinary school was founded in Lyon, France. At this time, divergence of the professions of farriery and veterinary medicine began to occur, with the appearance of the English word "veterinary" occurring in the late 18th century.[6] As both professions continued to evolve, each included hoof care within their respective missions.

However, by all accounts, farriery and veterinary medicine did not coexist in harmony and cooperation. Veterinary texts from the 19th and early 20th centuries reserve some of their harshest criticism for the farrier. Rebuttal is not easily found, as the farriers of the time were not inclined to publish their views. It should also be noted that farriery of the 19th and early 20th centuries was often a subset of black-smithing. The same arm and eye that worked the forge and anvil to create a horseshoe in the morning would craft a door hinge or plow shoe in the afternoon. For many veter-inary surgeons, the advantages of formal education and the freedom to concentrate on diseases of the horse, if not even solely on equine lameness, led to outspoken impatience with what they saw as inappropriate trimming and shoeing of both sound and lame horses. Readings of the texts from this era support this observation:

"The well-being of the best of animals is ever sacrificed to widespread ignorance and injustice. It is rare to find a shoeing-smith who possesses a really intelligent acquaintance with the wonderful structures of the 'horny box'; and we need not feel surprised that he should treat it much as he would a similar box of wood."[7]

"Bad and indifferent shoeing so frequently leads to diseases of the feet and in irregularities of gait which may render a horse unserviceable."[8]

"Now, what is there possessed by workers in iron, that they should know any more about diseases and their treatment than is possessed by a worker in wood?"[9]

"Without wishing to do injustice to our rural knights of the anvil, it is nevertheless a lamentable truth that these votaries of the buttress and drawing-knife are all the world over, so wedded to a number of traditionary [sic] practices, so heinous, so irrational, so prejudicial to the interests alike of the horse and his owner, that one might well be excused for wondering whether their mission were not to mar instead of to protect the marvelously perfect handiwork of the Creator. ... There is one instrument that I should like to see, if possible, omitted from the shoeing outfit of every farrier, and that is the drawing knife. If our blacksmiths would use their knives less and their heads more in the execution of their very important and by no means easy duty, our horses would be the better for it."[10]

This history is important and relevant to this discussion of therapeutic farriery. Although these criticisms may well have been accurate, they nonetheless did little to enfranchise the farrier into a cooperative effort with the veterinary surgeon to improve the health of the horse.

While tremendous progress has been made in advancing the knowledge base of both veterinarians and farriers, there still is much to be accomplished regarding the sharing of information, the dispassionate acceptance of constructive criticism, the acquisition of continuing education, and the nurturing of a strong sense of teamwork. For an equine practice to legitimately offer therapeutic farriery as a professional service, that service must be founded in individual competence and cooperation between veterinarian and farrier, with both striving to achieve a clear mission: the iden-tification of the definitive cause(s) of lameness and the application of the most appro-priate corrective farriery for the diagnosis(es) at hand.

DEFINITION

1. In modern equine practice, be it general or lameness-oriented, an understanding and implementation of therapeutic farriery are essential for success. So what is meant by "therapeutic farriery"? When and by whom was it first practiced? And under whose oversight does it most appropriately belong? This author considers therapeutic farriery as "the treatment of diseases or disorders of the equine limb by application of remedial methods and/or appliances to the digit." A colleague suggests it is the science and art of affecting or influencing the structures of the foot (S. O'Grady, personal communication, 2011).

Therapeutic farriery employs a broad range of treatments that extend from the simple removal of an inappropriate shoe (**Fig. 2**) to the use of sophisticated diagnostic imaging (**Fig. 3**) and construction of a custom appliance (**Fig. 4**). It is an important element in the delivery of health care to horses of all ages and disciplines and, thus, an essential professional service appropriately offered from any general and most specialty equine practices.

In a general sense, it is fair to say that therapeutic farriery was born when someone first attempted to correct a horse's hoof disorder or mitigate hoof pain, an event no doubt occurring many centuries ago. This basic concept of therapeutic farriery is the same today; what differs, of course, are the scientific and clinical knowledge bases and the sophisticated materials and instrumentation we now possess.

Finally, there may well be disagreement among practitioners and farriers as to when the definition of therapeutic farriery should—or should not—apply. For example, does it include measures believed to *prevent* both equine and human injury as well as maximize performance, such as the application of toe grabs to a race horse's shoes, heel calks for a stadium jumper, or borium cleats for winter trail riding? Might not these examples be better termed: *"performance farriery"*? Also, *ethical issues* may emerge

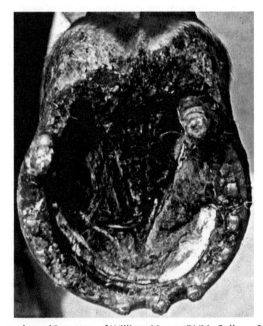

Fig. 2. Inappropriate shoe. (*Courtesy of* William Moyer, DVM, College Station, TX.)

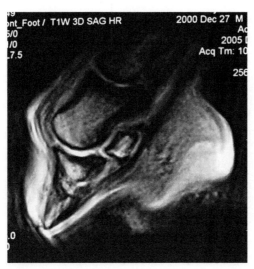

Fig. 3. Magnetic resonance image.

and must be addressed. Should the materials and methods of therapeutic farriery be applied to mitigate discomfort in a performance horse to keep it competing at the expense of facilitating the healing process with rest? Is pulling out all the stops on a severe and non-responsive case of laminitis considered "therapeutic farriery" or rather might it be a self-serving measure for the owner to satisfy personal emotional needs? Finally, while few would proclaim the use of trimming and appliances to sore the feet of some gaited horses to be therapeutic farriery (**Fig. 5**), this deplorable perversion of knowledge and skill persists today. In such cases, the real therapeutic farriery begins upon removal of the "package" and remedial trimming of the foot. Ultimately, such questions may be best answered on a case-by-case basis by the owner, farrier, and equine practitioner—as long as their top priority remains the health and welfare of the horse.

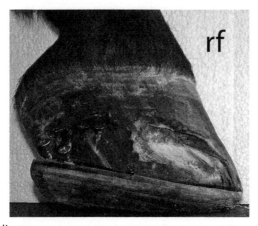

Fig. 4. Custom appliance.

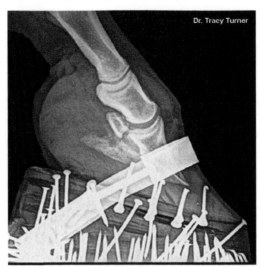

Fig. 5. Radiograph of Tennessee walking horse foot. (*Courtesy of* Dr Tracy A. Turner, DVM, Anoka Equine Veterinary Services, Elk River, MN.)

CURRENT STATUS OF EDUCATION IN THERAPEUTIC FARRIERY

Like most of the health professions, equine veterinary medicine has enjoyed an exponential advancement of knowledge and technology over the past two decades. These changes provide both challenges and opportunities to equine practitioners: the challenge to embrace the new science and technology and the opportunity to use them to improve equine health and welfare. In equine practice, these efforts are especially relevant in the prevention, diagnosis and management of orthopedic disease. Within this context, distal limb lamenesses are of predominant interest, especially those that involve the horse's digit. The digit is widely acknowledged to represent the site of the vast majority of equine lameness.[11] Thus, therapeutic farriery becomes a critically important element in the education of veterinary students as well as in the continuing education for established equine practitioners and farriers.

New veterinary school graduates appear to receive adequate and essential education regarding the pathophysiology and diagnostic imaging of the equine foot. Yet, it is the opinion of this author that they often begin practice with only a scant grasp of both the depth and scope of basic maintenance farriery, let alone therapeutic farriery. According to a recent survey: "VTH [veterinary teaching hospital] farrier services vary considerably in both nature and extent. The farriers' potential contributions to VTH operations are often recognized but not consistently exploited."[12] Additionally, this same survey compared and contrasted initial and continuing education requirements of American farriers and those in the United Kingdom:

"Of those attending farrier school (in the United States), many (33%) undertook a course lasting <3 months and only three (20%) completed a course lasting more than one year. Of those farriers undertaking apprenticeships, only 54% exceeded 2 years in duration. This compares unfavourably with the more rigorous professional farrier training requirements in other countries such as the UK where, for example, trainees must complete a four year apprenticeship with an Approved Training Farrier, during which they must undertake course work at farrier school as well as a diploma examination. Additionally, only one (5%) VTH farrier was required to attend any form of continuing education, a source of concern when one considers the farrier and veterinary professions' growing understanding of both theoretical and practical farriery such as hoof form and function or the growing number of polymer products available for hoof capsule repair. By comparison, obligatory continuing education attendance has been required of all UK farriers since 2008."[12]

Inadequate farriery education and experience may result in substandard or even contraindicated therapeutic farriery prescriptions and farrier care, a consequence that is obviously contrary not only to the horse's best interests but also to the professional growth and stature of the veterinarian and farrier. Furthermore, an experienced farrier may well rightfully resist, if not reject, working with a veterinarian whose prescription for therapeutic farriery is clearly inappropriate. Various equine veterinary[13] and farriery[14] associations in North America and abroad[15,16] are making significant and effective efforts to address the need for better education in this important area. For example, the American Association of Equine Practitioners Farriery Short Course for veterinary students sends a Certified Journeyman Farrier and an American Association of Equine Practitioners member equine practitioner to the veterinary schools for a day-long lecture and hands-on farriery demonstration. This program promotes the veterinarian/farrier relationship, focuses on hoof biomechanics and lower limb anatomy, and demonstrates the different types of horse shoes and their applications.

Within the venue of continuing education for equine practitioners, excellent opportunities to advance one's understanding of and clinical competence in therapeutic farriery are increasingly available. With presentations by respected experts from farriery, clinical veterinary practice, and the basic sciences, professional development in this essential area has never been more readily achievable. The importance of equine practitioners achieving and maintaining competence in this essential area of equine practice cannot be overstated.

For farriers, excellent continuing education opportunities are now more numerous than ever before and are offered by universities, veterinary associations, private veterinary practices, and industry manufacturers and suppliers. Quality continuing education events that enjoin both equine practitioners and farriers are the most powerful means of encouraging communication and cooperation between the two professions. Such events strengthen this historic partnership that is based on mutual respect and understanding. It is the essential foundation on which the successful practice of therapeutic farriery is built. It is this author's opinion that quality continuing education opportunities for farriers are greatly underutilized; it is also this author's experience that it often takes only some encouragement from equine practitioners to motivate the farriers with whom they work to attend. Such efforts can stimulate professional growth for both parties and result in better care for the horses on which they work.

THE PARTNERSHIP

The working partnership between veterinarians and farriers has endured for well over two centuries. Like any long-term human relationship, it enjoys periods of harmony as well as more difficult times. This is not surprising when one considers that both parties, while equally sharing the goals of helping the horse and earning a living, often come from sharply different backgrounds by the time they are bent over the hoof and debating what to do next. Additionally, both are likely to be working in a "fishbowl" environment, in full view of owners, trainers, grooms, clients (past, present, and future), and other farriers and veterinarians. Such exposure demands that both the veterinarian and the farrier behave and speak in a professional manner if a true partnership is to evolve.

The Farrier

The farrier lives her or his working life in intimate physical contact with the horse. Owners expect their farrier to attend on a regular schedule and to show little sign of suffering when foul weather or fractious horses prevail. Pain, at least periodically, is a given and is simply part of the job. Owners rightly expect their farrier to be a horseman, capable of quietly working without inciting the slightest trace of anxiety in the beast—despite the pounding of steel on steel, the smoke cloud of a hot fit, and the driving of nails just a sliver distant from sensitive tissue. In addition to being able to forge steel shoes out of bar stock, the competent farrier must possess the knowledge and skills necessary to properly select from an ever-growing list of synthetics and effectively apply their choice when needed. A "normal" horse is not only the best possible outcome but, most important, the only acceptable outcome to many owners. In other words, when shoeing a sound horse, the stature of a farrier can at best stay unchanged, if not actually deteriorate. The International Hall of Fame farrier Jackie Thompson once stated: "You can shoe the top racehorse and no one will know; let one shoe come off, and its international news."[17] Because the farrier's vocation is physically demanding and technically challenging, most are justly proud of their work and often quickly suspect of any outside criticism, regardless of how constructive it was meant to be. This tendency is even more likely to appear when the farrier's years or depth of experience clearly exceeds that of the veterinarian. As the farrier sees the horse on a regular basis, he or she is often the first to observe changes in the hoof capsule, the horse's overall comfort while standing for farriery, or the earliest indications of foot pain. Such observations are an invaluable and often unwritten record that the equine practitioner is well-advised to access. However, such a professional partnership requires mutual respect, trust, and striving for a common goal.

The Veterinarian

While highly educated in a broad range of clinical sciences, new graduates are often inexperienced and underinformed in the field of farriery, be it basic maintenance or therapeutic. Many internship opportunities reportedly still offer scant preparation for solo management of therapeutic farriery cases. There is often an internal conflict within the veterinarian between an awareness of his/her own lack of experience versus the pressure to appear as the dominant professional—that is, "the doctor." For many, this conflict translates into forcing the farrier—rightly or wrongly—into a subordinate position and can create a barrier to building an effective working relationship. It has been suggested that a useful guideline for young or inexperienced practitioners is that "it is a good idea to be respectful in all discussions with people who carry hammers & bend iron for a living"![18]

That said, the equine practitioner, not the farrier, holds the keys to discovering the definitive diagnosis in most lamenesses. Careful taking of the history; accurate and thorough recording of the medical record; deliberate observations, palpations, and manipulations; sequential and careful applications of diagnostic anesthesia; and select diagnostic imaging studies are essential components of most lameness examinations. In total, these are the purview and primary responsibility of the equine practitioner, not the farrier. It must also be remembered at all times that the lame limb is attached to a horse! It does little good to practice therapeutic farriery for laminitis in a vacuum, thus failing to identify the insulin-resistant patient, the horse with equine Cushing's disease, or the client's recent purchase of black walnut shavings for bedding.

Finally, it cannot be overstated that it is the obligation of the veterinarian to acquire and maintain a working understanding of the elements of both basic and therapeutic farriery if he or she is to work effectively with the farrier and offer a valid service to the client for their horse. In this author's experience and opinion, the foundation of this understanding consists of the principles of clinical examination[19], proper hoof trimming[20] and the biomechanics of the equine limb.[21] If the veterinarian finds that he or she can not acquire and maintain this understanding successfully, then the patient should be referred to an equine practitioner who can do so—just as one would refer a patient to meet any other clinical need.

CONFLICT AND RESOLUTION

The establishment of a productive and lasting veterinary–farrier partnership can be inhibited by:

- Failure of either professional to perform with competence and integrity
- Failure of either professional to understand the demands placed upon the other
- A lack of respect by one professional for the knowledge and/or experience of the other
- Criticism—deserved or otherwise—expressed indiscreetly
- Failure of either professional to communicate fully and accurately and in a timely manner

As in any relationship, respect and trust are earned over time. It is not enough for either the veterinarian or the farrier to do their respective jobs well but in isolation. If the patient is to benefit, both parties must communicate freely and be mutually supportive of each other's efforts.

For the veterinarian, there should be no tolerance for anything less than the most accurate diagnosis that can be achieved under the circumstances; this, after all, will be the compass used to guide the farrier and to determine further veterinary care. One cannot expect a best outcome with a wrong diagnosis, no matter how good the therapeutic farriery. Achieving an accurate diagnosis requires examining the case in a stepwise, thorough manner. A common violation of this approach is to leap to diagnostic imaging on nothing more than a hunch. The "instant gratification" associated with today's digital imaging technologies, their technical excellence notwithstanding, makes such an expedient approach to lameness diagnosis an everyday temptation. "Dependence upon imaging modalities without precise localization of the source of the problems has, at times, has been miss-leading as well as a waste of money."[22] In many cases, the most important diagnostic instruments may well be a fever thermometer and a hoof tester. Conclusively locating the source of pain *before* moving to diagnostic imaging should be a goal of every lameness examination and this approach will win the respect and cooperation of the farrier. Including the farrier in the examination process, explaining the findings, and requesting the farrier's input not only are helpful relationship-builders, but they very often result in valuable insights and information gained.

It is the veterinarian's responsibility to acquire and interpret radiographs. The sharing of the radiographic image and interpretation with the farrier is an appropriate and important step in the therapeutic farriery process. However, it is this author's opinion that it is clearly unethical to facilitate or encourage a farrier to possess or utilize radiographic equipment and/or interpret radiographs without direct veterinary oversight. This serious breach of ethics is also a violation of most—if not all—state practice acts. It introduces unprofessional behavior into therapeutic farriery and does a disservice to the equine practitioner, the client, the farrier, and—most important—the horse. Finally, compliance with acceptable radiation safety standards is unlikely to occur without professional training and regulatory oversight.

The farrier's good works should be acknowledged, not only to him or her but to the owner as well; when criticism is appropriate, it should be expressed privately and professionally. However, it must be conceded that in some instances, a positive and productive veterinary–farrier relationship simply may not be possible. In such a case, for the welfare of the horse, the dilemma should be discussed frankly with the owner so that alternatives can be promptly enacted.

THE CLIENT

Increasingly, veterinarians work for horse owners rather than horsemen. Some cases involving therapeutic farriery will remain open cases for months or years. Horsemen understand this scenario but non-horsemen usually do not. Thus, it is essential to advise and inform the owner, as clearly as possible, regarding the estimated duration of therapy, its possible financial costs, and the patient's prognosis. In many cases, this information changes over time and requires ongoing communication with an owner. For performance horses, the equine practitioner must have a working knowledge of that horse's intended use including any restrictions or requirements (practical or regulatory) that may affect treatment options. For example, has the therapeutic farriery increased the withers height of a pony hunter beyond its official United States Equestrian Federation designation? Has a therapeutic farriery device caused the toe length of an Arabian to exceed the regulatory limit? Will the need for traction devices in a pulling horse be contraindicated from a therapeutic perspective? It is unwise to assume that such considerations are obvious to many of today's owners. The veterinarian and farrier can avoid troubling unintended consequences by remaining conscious of intended use limitations.

While some cases utilizing therapeutic farriery may enjoy a relatively quick and successful conclusion, many take more time and may result in a downgrade in the horse's athletic career. One should not assume that these issues are clear to the owner or that the owner possesses the resources necessary—or the will to commit such resources—to support long-term therapeutic farriery. Failure to educate the client can damage the welfare of the patient, professional reputations, and long-standing relationships among farriers, owners, and veterinarians. An example of this problem is often the horse with chronic laminitis, a disease that is expensive to manage, is treated by means with little to no solid evidence-based efficacy data and with no certainty of a positive outcome.[23] Further complicating the effort to educate the owner in such difficult cases is the abundance of nonsense readily available from the Internet and proffered by many from within the horse world; it is nearly impossible to name an equine lameness for which someone does not have a cure or knows someone who does. The equine practitioner must remain the source of credible information for the owner. Additionally, when a medical insurance claim has been made, the veterinarian must accurately complete and submit all requested reports to the insurer in a timely manner.

Finally, a reality of human nature is a tendency to place blame and many owners of lame horses are inclined to do so; in the absence of compelling evidence to support the claim, "it is unethical for veterinarians and farriers to indicate to owners that had someone instituted a particular therapy at a particular time in the course of the disease that the horse could have had a better outcome."[24]

THE HORSE'S HEALTH CARE TEAM

As a patient who cannot represent its own interests, a horse is totally dependent on the stewardship of its caregivers. In cases of lameness, these caregivers are the owner, the farrier, and the equine practitioner. In many cases, the horse's trainer will be an active member of the team, as well. In some cases, the trainer will act on behalf of the owner. As such, the trainer must as well be kept informed and can provide valuable oversight and reports between visits. Each of these individuals is most effective, and the horse benefits most, when they act as a team (**Fig. 6**). To do so, they must each benefit from mutual understanding and clear and timely communication. These goals are best met if the veterinarian and farrier engage in frequent and open dialogues and avoid acting on assumptions regarding the patient or its owner. Competent care involves attention to everything from scheduling the next appointment and who will attend to specifics of trimming, shoeing and ancillary therapy. If there is to be client-administered aftercare, the details of such must be clearly spelled out in writing. However, it must be remembered that the trainer is *not* the owner; assuming that the trainer can and will always accurately portray the status of a case to the owner invites misunderstanding and conflict. It remains the equine veterinarian's responsibility to ensure that the owner is kept appropriately informed in a timely manner. A good rule of thumb to practice is: *Allow no surprises!*

In addition to maximizing the quality of care the horse enjoys, a team approach is also very effective in building client appreciation as well as minimizing any risk of misunderstanding, negative feelings, and subsequent legal action.

COMMUNICATIONS AND MEDICAL RECORDS

It is likely that most relationships break down from too little—rather than too much—communication. The successful veterinary–farrier relationship is highly dependent on clear, accurate, and timely communication. An essential part of this communication is the proper use of applicable terms.[25,26] Appropriate terminology minimizes risks of

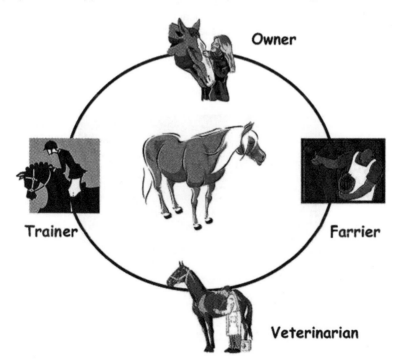

Owner

Trainer

Farrier

Veterinarian

Fig. 6. The equine health care team.

errors in patient care and fosters effective communication with owners. Equine practitioners and farriers should challenge each other's use of terms so that clear understanding and accuracy can prevail.

Satisfied owners usually want to be included in the professional care of their horses and expect to be kept informed in a timely manner regarding their horses' care. Such information can include:

- Updates on current status
- Proposed diagnostic and treatment plans
- Estimates of anticipated costs
- Changes in prognosis

Effective communication to clients achieves two essential goals: it conveys the value of services and it avoids the surprise of unexpected fees. It cannot be assumed that clients always understand and appreciate the scope and depth of professional services unless they are explained. Client understanding and appreciation are achieved when both the veterinarian and farrier consciously make themselves the owner's primary source for education.

Medical records and communication are areas that are greatly facilitated by modern technology. Cell phones, e-mail, portable printers, digital cameras, and digital diagnostic imaging modalities (radiography, ultrasonography and thermal imaging) all facilitate the rapid acquisition and transmission of information relevant to therapeutic farriery.

Acquisition of an accurate medical history is the essential first step in the therapeutic farriery process. This can be easily captured with a hand-held recorder; an even more efficient means is a hand-held recorder that automatically converts voice to printed text and allows for e-mail transmission (eg, Dragon Dictation, Nuance Communications, Burlington, Massachusetts). This technology lends itself well to real-time recording of findings for entry into the medical record.

Image capture and archiving is an essential tool in therapeutic farriery. A simple digital camera with a minimum of five megapixels, a macro lens setting, and video capture capability is invaluable for acquisition of both still and motion images. Any of the basic image manipulation software programs will allow quick enhancement and labeling of images (**Fig. 7**) as well as conversion to a variety of formats for

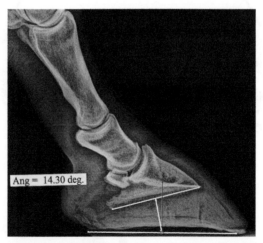

Fig. 7. Image enhancement and labeling. (*Courtesy of* Robert H. Kraybill, DVM, Cumberland Valley Equine Services, Carlisle, PA.)

transmission or storage. For ambulatory practitioners, traveling with a laptop computer allows immediate access to case histories and diagnostic images, image examples of digit anatomy (**Fig. 8**), and therapeutic farriery applications (**Fig. 9**) for farrier and client education and for completing reporting templates. Word processing software allows reporting templates to be built and stored electronically in pdf format. Data entry is minimized and the insertion of relevant images completes the report. Communication between owner, veterinarian, and farrier can be achieved via e-mailing or, in ambulatory practice, printing out a hard copy of the document (**Fig. 10**). For example, when radiography is included in a prepurchase examination, a "farrier report" (**Fig. 11**) that shows dorsopalmar and lateromedial views of the feet provides the farrier with a valuable benchmark. Finally, especially helpful to this author in client and farrier communications has been the interactive software program The Equine Distal Limb (**Fig. 12**) (Glass Horse Project, LLC, Athens, GA, USA).[27] Carried to cases in a laptop computer, it greatly facilitates demonstration of equine distal limb anatomy and, thus, explanation of pathology and proposed farriery.

The creation of a timely, accurate, and ongoing medical record complete with relevant images is an essential element of good practice. It can also be an invaluable asset should legal actions or insurance challenges arise.

Expert Consultation

Equine practitioners are fortunate to enjoy the presence of farriery experts within both the veterinary and farriery communities. One should become familiar with these individuals and their published works as they are valuable resources. Most welcome questions and are willing to consult on cases. Many experts have websites that offer excellent and practical advice on specific topics. Establishing a network with select individuals adds a valuable dimension to practices offering therapeutic farriery. The details of any professional consultation should be recorded in the medical record and shared with the client to clearly convey value and to encourage client compliance with the therapeutic plan.

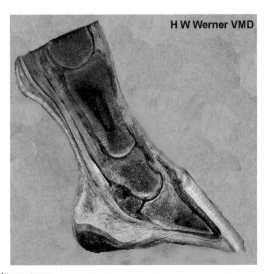

Fig. 8. Equine digit anatomy.

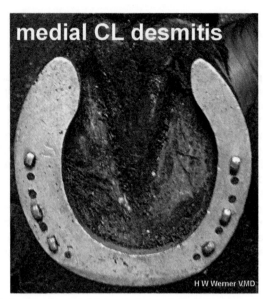

Fig. 9. Therapeutic farriery for distal interphalangeal medial collateral desmitis.

WHAT WE KNOW VERSUS WHAT WE THINK WE KNOW

While the bank of knowledge regarding the form and function of the equine foot is rich with information, it is important to realize that only some of this information is founded on solid evidence. Many of the axioms by which practitioners and farriers work daily remain based on their own case experiences, anecdotes from a colleague or mentor, or simply pronouncements that have been stated and restated so often that they assume an air of established truth.

Over the past several decades, veterinarians have witnessed radical changes in what is considered correct interpretation of the radiographic appearance of the navicular bone and of the "proper" way to trim the acutely laminitic foot. These changes resulted from extensive laboratory and clinical studies in pathophysiology, the effects of various farriery applications, and the development of sophisticated diagnostic imaging modalities such as digital and computed radiography, computed tomography, and magnetic resonance imaging. Even with today's knowledge, farriers and veterinarians continue to question what much of what we "know" really means.

Evidence-based data are difficult and costly to obtain in equine research. Most research into equine distal limb biomechanics and the effects of farriery techniques has been performed either in vitro or on sound horses. While such research models provide thought-provoking and valuable information, its applicability in treating the lame horse remains unproved.[28] This dilemma was addressed in 2003 by the editors of *Equine Veterinary Journal* in an editorial entitled "Clinical Evidence: An Avenue to Evidence-Based Medicine"[29] and again in the same journal in 2009, under the title of "Case Reports versus Evidence-Based Medicine (EBM)."[30]

If therapeutic farriery is to evolve to be as effective as possible, practitioners and farriers alike must consistently challenge traditionally held theories, conventional wisdom, and, in fact, their own clinical experiences. They must not just evaluate published material on its subject matter, author, or application to their own particular needs but rather seek to understand the strength of the scientific and/or clinical

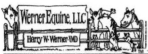

Since 1979 – Providing veterinary care that improves the health and welfare of the Horse

FARRIER RADIOGRAPHY REPORT - farrier, Danny Dunson

OWNER: Harris, Thomas   **PATIENT: STRETCH**   **DATE: 4-4-2009**

DIAGNOSTIC PLAN: Digital radiography was performed to evaluate right fore foot lameness.

IMAGING TARGETS AND FINDINGS:

- **left fore foot:** normal.

- **right fore foot:** dorsal rotation of P3; osteolysis of dorsal tip of right 3rd phalanx.

INTERPRETATION OF FINDINGS: chronic laminitis of right fore foot.

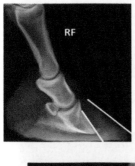
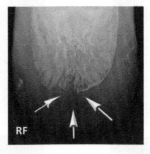
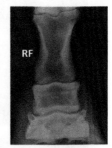
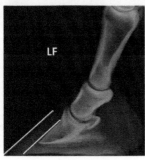
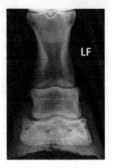

Attending Veterinarian: Harry W. Werner VMD

Member, American Association of Equine Practitioners   1/1

20 Godard Road P.O. Box 5 North Granby, CT 06060   Tel (860) 653-5088   Fax (860) 653-5080   www.wernerequine.com

Fig. 10. Radiography report.

evidence on which its conclusions are drawn. Likewise, the therapeutic farriery marketplace offers no shortage of fads, both intellectual and material. Veterinarians and farriers must do battle with those who would have others believe that they alone possess knowledge of the only proper farrier techniques or proprietary rights to the

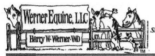

Since 1979 – Providing veterinary care that improves the health and welfare of the Horse

FARRIER PREPURCHASE EXAMINATION RADIOGRAPHY REPORT

OWNER: Collins, Helen   PATIENT: CLEO   DATE: 8-1-11

DIAGNOSTIC PLAN: Radiography was performed as part of prepurchase examination and as resource for farriery. No lameness was noted during the examination.

INTERPRETATION: sheared lateral heel at each fore foot; no palmar angles.

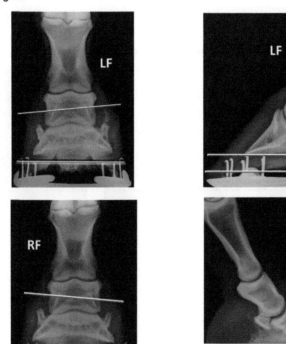

Attending Veterinarian: Harry W. Werner VMD

Member, American Association of Equine Practitioners   1/1

20 Godard Road   P.O. Box 5   North Granby, CT 06060   Tel (860) 653-5088   Fax (860) 653-5080   www.wernerequine.com

Fig. 11. Farrier report.

only correct therapeutic hoof appliances. The professional marketing of sound science and credible clinical reports is essential for the practice of therapeutic farriery to evolve and its practitioners to grow professionally. However, the marketing of unsubstantiated theories or devices guaranteed to cure shows a lack of integrity and has no place in the practice of good equine medicine.

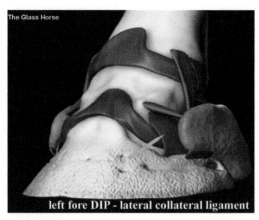
The Glass Horse

left fore DIP - lateral collateral ligament

Fig. 12. The Equine Distal Limb.

SUMMARY

Providing therapeutic farriery in an equine practice is an opportunity to join and strengthen a centuries-old relationship between veterinarians and farriers, to increase a veterinary practice's case load of lameness diagnosis and treatment, and to positively affect the quality of the lives of many horses. It is a discipline that joins art with science and enjoys an ancient history while using the most recent advances in science and technology.

A relationship based on mutual trust and respect is essential between the farrier and the veterinarian. Clear, correct, and timely communication enhances this relationship and the quality of patient care.

The horse deserves to be considered in its entirety, not simply as a lame limb. The equine practitioner and the farrier both owe their patients a serious commitment to remaining current in their professional education.

The client deserves honest and understandable explanations regarding diagnosis, proposed treatments, prognosis, and anticipated costs. This requires taking the time to communicate with the client verbally as well as providing imaging reports, client education summaries, clearly written aftercare instructions, periodic case updates, and timely cost estimates. A client who understands the case at hand and the challenges facing the farrier and veterinarian will become a valuable member of the horse's health care team.

In the future, it is this author's hope that veterinary educators will find ways to adjust today's already full curricula to embrace increased instruction in both basic and therapeutic farriery and that the opportunities for professional development of both farriers and equine practitioners will continue to grow. Finally, it is hoped that research will continue to produce knowledge, techniques, and materials relevant and applicable to therapeutic farriery. Given their millennia of sacrifice and service to mankind, our horses deserve no less.

REFERENCES

1. International Museum of the Horse. What we theorize—when and where did domestication occur? Available at: http://imh.org/history-of-the-horse/legacy-of-the-horse/the-domestication-of-the-horse/what-we-theorize-when-and-where-did-domestication-occur.html. Accessed March 15, 2012.

2. Gemoll W. Hyginus gromaticus liber de munitionibus castrorum. 21:1879 Available at: http://archive.org/details/liberdemunitioni00hygiuoft. Accessed April 10, 2012.

3. Online Etymology Dictionary. Available at: http://www.etymonline.com/index.php?allowed_in_frame=0&search=farrier&searchmode=none. Accessed May 5, 2012.

4. Holmes OW. The common law. Boston: Little, Brown, and Co; 1881.

5. Bullock F. Notes on the early history of the veterinary surgeon in England. Proc R Soc Med 1929;22(5):627–33.

6. Available at: http://www.etymonline.com/index.php?allowed_in_frame=0&search=veterinarian&searchmode=none. Accessed March 15, 2012.

7. Armatage G. The horse: management in health and disease. Frederick Warneand Co; 1893. p. 260.

8. Adams JW. Diseases of the horse. Washington, DC: US Department of Agriculture; 1907. p. 559.

9. McClure R. Diseases of the American horse and cattle and sheep. John E. Potter and Co; 1870. p. 90.

10. Dickson W. Diseases of the horse. Washington, DC: US Department of Agriculture; 1890. p. 530–2.

11. Moyer W. Clinical examination of the equine foot. Vet Clin North Am Equine Pract 1989;5(1):29–46.

12. Kirker-Head CA, Krane G. Farrier services at veterinary teaching hospitals in the USA. Equine Vet Educ 2010;22:519–25.

13. American Association of Equine Practitioners. Farrier short course. Available at: http://www.aaep.org/farrier_short_course.htm. Accessed March 15, 2012.

14. American Farriers Journal. International Hoof Care Summit. Available at: www.americanfarriers.com.

15. BEVA. British Equine Veterinary Association. Foot and remedial farriery course. Available at: www.beva.org.uk.

16. Worshipful Company of Farriers. Available at: http://www.wcf.org.uk/continuing_professional_development. Accessed March 5, 2012.

17. Norma S. The K.I.S.S. approach for shoeing the racehorse. Baltimore (MD): AAEP 56th Annual Convention Farriery Program, December 8, 2010.

18. Merriam JG. The role and importance of farriery in equine veterinary practice. Vet Clin North Am Equine Pract 2003;19(2):273–83.

19. Moyer W. Clinical Examination and interpretation of the equine foot. Vet Clin North Am Equine Pract 1989;5(1):29–48.

20. O'Grady S, Poupard D. Proper Physiologic Horseshoeing. Vet Clin North Am Equine Pract 2003;19(2):333–52.

21. Parks A. Form and function of the equine digit. Vet Clin North Am Equine Pract 2003;19(2):273–84.

22. Moyer W. Practical Aspects of Diagnosing Lameness in Horses: A Suggested Procedure for Performing the Physical and Motion Examination. Costa Rica: AAEP 12th Annual Resort Symposium. January 24-26, 2010.

23. Moyer W, Schumacher J. Chronic laminitis: considerations for the owner and prevention of misunderstandings. AAEP Proc 2000;46:60.

24. Moyer W, Schumacher J. Chronic laminitis: considerations for the owner and prevention of misunderstandings. Proceedings. 46th Annual American Association of Equine Practitioners Convention 2000;46:61.

25. O'Grady SE. Podiatry terminology. Equine Vet Educ 2007;19(5):263–71.

26. Parks AH, Mair TS. Laminitis: a call for unified terminology. Equine Vet Educ 2009; 21(2):102–6.

27. Glass Horse Project LLC. Available at: http://www.3dglasshorse.com/default.asp. Accessed May 5, 2012.
28. Eliashar E. An evidence-based assessment of the biomechanical effects of the common shoeing and farriery techniques. Vet Clin North Am Equine Pract 2007;23(2):425–42.
29. Rossdale PD, Jeffcott LB, Holmes MA. Clinical evidence: an avenue to evidence-based medicine. Equine Vet J 2003;35(7):634–5.
30. Rossdale PD. Case reports versus evidence-based medicine (EBM). Equine Vet J 2009;41(4):322–3.

The Biomechanics of the Equine Foot as it Pertains to Farriery

Ehud Eliashar, BSc, DVM, MRCVS

KEYWORDS

- Horse • Shoes • Farriery • Biomechanics

KEY POINTS

- The basic principle creating the lameness that is observe in the horse is the attempt the horse makes to unload the painful limb.
- Trimming results in significant increase in contact surface area, characterized by increased uniformity of wall contact, increase in the contact of the peripheral sole, and appearance of contact of the frog and bars.
- Heel wedges do not unload the heels, hence it is likely that their use in horses with collapsed heels has to be time limited or the condition may worsen.
- There is still a significant deficit in veterinary knowledge regarding the effects of shoeing and farriery techniques on clinically affected lame horses, or horses with identified clinical conditions, and comparisons of unshod and shod horses are rare.

INTRODUCTION

The function of the hoof can be affected by means other than farriery manipulations, such as changes in riding pattern or daily exercise, pregnancy, diet, and housing. The hoof has the ability to respond to these changes in 2 ways. The first, provided by its structural characteristics, is its natural tolerance of the mechanical challenges it is exposed to. The second mechanism is the hoof's ability to respond over time by adaptation, most obviously with changes in growth rate and shape.[1]

Although the original reason for applying shoes to horses was to protect against excessive wear,[2] over the years, countless types of shoes and farriery techniques have been developed not only as a therapeutic aid to treat lameness but also to maintain or enhance functionality.[3]

The past 3 decades have provided equine veterinarians and farriers with new information relating to limb biomechanics and the effects of various farriery methods. Obtaining much of this information became possible with advances in technology and the availability of powerful computers, forceplates, pressure mats, motion analysis systems, gyroscopes, and accelerometers. These advances then allowed finer

St Albans, Hertfordshire, UK
E-mail address: ehud@eliashar.com

Vet Clin Equine 28 (2012) 283–291
http://dx.doi.org/10.1016/j.cveq.2012.06.001
0749-0739/12/$ – see front matter © 2012 Elsevier Inc. All rights reserved.

analysis of the effects of various shoeing interventions in prospective biomechanical studies.

This article describes the principles of foot biomechanics and how they are affected by some of the more common farriery and shoeing techniques. More detailed information regarding the evidence behind the use of these techniques was published in a previous issue of this publication.[4]

THE PRINCIPLES OF FOOT BIOMECHANICS

The stride can be divided into 2 phases. Flight phase is the part of stride during which the limb is airborne and has no contact with the ground. The second phase is the stance phase, during which the foot is in contact with the ground and the limb is therefore subjected to an external impact force by the ground. This external impact is termed the ground reaction force (GRF), the magnitude of which depends on the horse's weight, speed of movement,[5] and the surface on which the horse moves,[6] and it is considered the most critical part of the stance phase for developing injuries of the musculoskeletal system.[7] For ease of mathematical calculations, the GRF is considered to act at a single point under the foot defined as the point of zero moment (PZM) or point of force (PoF).[8,9] However, this point is not positioned directly under the center of rotation of the distal interphalangeal (DIP) joint. Rather, it is positioned horizontally, away from the center of rotation of the joint, which creates a lever, or what is referred to as a moment arm. The action of the GRF and its moment arm creates a torque; that is, a force that produces or tends to produce rotation or torsion. This torque is the extending moment of the DIP joint (**Fig. 1**).

The extending moment of the DIP joint is balanced by an equal flexing moment generated by the deep digital flexor tendon (DDFT). Another moment arm is created by the tendon running over the navicular bone.[10] As a result of the deviation of the

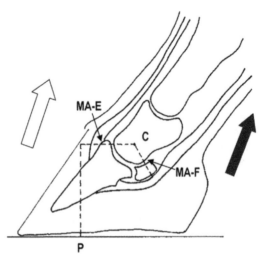

Fig. 1. The various moments acting to extend and flex the DIP joint. C, center of rotation of the DIP joint; MA-E, extending moment arm of the DIP joint; MA-F, flexing moment arm of the DIP joint; P, point of zero moment. White arrow, extending moment of the DIP joint; black arrow, flexing moment of the DIP joint. (*From* Eliashar E. An evidence-based assessment of the biomechanical effects of the common shoeing and farriery techniques. Vet Clin North Am Equine Pract 2007;23:425–42; with permission.)

DDFT around the navicular bone, during the stance phase of the stride the tendon compresses the navicular bone, with a force that is proportional not only to the DDFT force but also to the angle of deviation of the DDFT around the bone.[11–13] By measuring the surface area of the flexor cortex of the navicular bone, the stress imposed on the bone by the DDFT throughout stance can be calculated.[13,14]

Toward the end of stance, because the heels are gradually unloading at this time, the PZM moves toward the toe. When the PZM reaches the toe, the DIP joint moment arm cannot increase further because the moment arm can go no farther forward on the hoof. As a result, the extending moment decreases in line with the reducing GRF. At this stage, the flexing moment exceeds the extending moment, and the DIP joint flexes; that is, the heels leave the ground. This period at the terminal part of the stance phase is called breakover. During breakover, the time from heel-off to toe-off, the heel rotates around the toe.[11,15]

CONFORMATION AND BALANCE

Both conformation and balance are frequently mentioned in reference to the shape and size of the distal limb and the spatial relations between its different elements,[16,17] and it is therefore important to distinguish between them. Conformation describes the general shape, size, and static relations of the distal limb.[16] Balance embraces both shape and function of the foot in relation to the ground, as well as to skeletal structures of the limb, both at rest and at exercise.[18] Each foot should have a conformation that maximizes its mechanical efficiency, and, when such conformation is thought to have been achieved by trimming the foot, the foot is said to be balanced.[17]

For years, veterinarians and farriers have been trying to define the ideal hoof balance that a normal sound horse should have. At present, the debate is far from reaching a unified conclusion. Several techniques have therefore been described for assessing hoof balance. Geometric balance is defined as the attempt to make the hoof as symmetric as possible around its sagittal solar plane, which occupies a prescribed position in relation to the rest of the foot. Dynamic balance is defined as the conformation that allows the foot to contact the ground in a prescribed pattern.[17] Techniques such as Duckett's dot and the natural balance trim assess balance in relation to a reference point or a formula.

Regardless of the technique used to achieve the desired shape, it is widely accepted that conformation and balance of both hoof and distal limb, and the interaction with movement, trimming, shoeing, and ground surfaces, are important factors in equine hoof and distal limb health and performance.[19]

GROWTH AND WEAR

The processes of hoof growth and wear should be balanced. This balance allows an unshod horse to maintain the shape and size of its feet, although the size and shape are directly influenced by the characteristics of the surface on which the horse lives, and the friction between it and the sole.[17,20] However, in the domesticated shod horse, friction occurs between the expanding heel and the shoe, inducing greater wear at the heel compared with that of the toe, which, over time, results in changes in hoof balance.[21,22]

Unshod sound horses kept in pasture develop a solar surface that has a weight-bearing load distribution of either a 4-point or 3-point pattern.[17] When standing on a deformable surface, load distribution in these horses is principally solar, and an abrasive surface causes a rapid change in the solar pattern of load distribution, with loss of the 3-point or 4-point patterns, and increased contact of the peripheral wall, bars, and frog.[17] It therefore seems that friction is responsible for the shape of the unshod feet, which may further suggest that a more uniform distribution is perhaps more natural and potentially more beneficial.[1]

As the hoof grows in the shod horse, the dorsal hoof angle typically becomes shallower, the PZM moves in a palmar/plantar direction, and the hoof rolls in a more lateral direction, especially in the hind limbs.[21] Furthermore, hoof growth results in extension of the DIP joint, whereas there is no significant change in the angle at the proximal interphalangeal (PIP) joint.[22] However, these changes seem to have no effect on the force and stress exerted by the DDFT on the navicular bone, possibly as a result of a compensatory mechanism that is not understood.[23]

FARRIERY MANIPULATIONS

The basic principle creating lameness in the horse is the attempt the horse makes to unload the painful limb. In a similar way, corrective shoeing and farriery techniques attempt to unload a specific site, and/or to shorten the duration that the site is bearing weight. Among others, these manipulations attempt to induce change in toe length, the position or shape of the toe, change in heel or toe height, or change in ground contact area. Any of these can be achieved by trimming, use of a special shoe, incorporation of a wedge, or any combination. Many of these manipulations, especially in the sagittal plane, have received much attention from veterinarians and farriers, mainly as a result of the widely suggested involvement of such changes in the pathophysiology of many foot ailments, such as conditions involving the navicular apparatus.[24,25]

CHANGES IN GROUND CONTACT AREA

Trimming results in significant increase in contact surface area, characterized by increased uniformity of wall contact, increase in the contact of the peripheral sole, and appearance of contact of the frog and bars.[17] Furthermore, it is suggested that trimming promotes a more even load distribution,[19] because it decreases the variability between contralateral limbs and hence loading of the structures of the caudal hoof.[21]

Egg-bar shoes are probably the most common farriery technique used to increase the ground contact area with shoes. The rationales for applying these shoes to increase the ground contact area include an attempt to bring about a more correct weight distribution and to provide extra support to the heel.[26,27] Egg-bar shoes decrease maximal extension of the DIP joint at heel-off and they seem to stabilize the hoof in the transverse plane.[28] Furthermore, these shoes cause a negligible reduction in the maximal strain of the DDFT but also seem to increase the strain of the suspensory ligament (SL),[27] and prevent the heels from sinking into the ground on a sand track.[28,29] In sound horses, egg-bar shoes do not have any effect on the force exerted by the DDFT on the navicular bone,[12] but, in some clinically affected horses, mainly those with collapsed heel conformation, significant reduction in the force and stress exerted on the navicular bone is observed.[30] It seems therefore that egg-bar shoes have some effects on unloading the distal limb.[29]

CHANGE IN TOE POSITION OR LENGTH

The notion that creating a longer toe by trimming feet with a more acute angle has any significant effect on stride length has long been refuted.[31,32] Furthermore, toe length or angle does not affect the duration of stance phase, but, in the barefooted horse, breakover duration is significantly prolonged with a longer toe.[12] Moving the toe position back using shoes with different toe profiles significantly shortens the moment arm of the GRF on the DIP joint but does not alter the duration of breakover or the force exerted on the navicular bone.[11]Rocker-toe, rolled-toe, or square-toe shoes similarly have no significant effect on the duration of breakover in comparison with conventional plain steel shoes.[15,33] Rolled-toe shoes are suggested to reduce peak DIP joint moment by 14%, allowing smoother and more gradual hoof movement[34]; however, there is no clinical evidence that the use of this type of shoe is ideal for every horse.

CHANGE IN HEEL/TOE HEIGHT

The immediate effect of elevating 1 side of the hoof, for example with the use of a wedge, is displacement of the PZM toward the elevated side.[9] Although stance duration is not affected by application of a wedge,[9,28,35] the wedge induces not only a higher load on the elevated side[35] and a change to the pattern of hoof impact,[12] but it also affects multiple other structures of the foot. Heel wedge delays unloading of the heel,[9,28,35] shortening breakover by about 1.5% of stance duration.[35]

It is generally accepted that increasing heel height induces flexion of the DIP and PIP joints and increases intra-articular pressure of the DIP joint.[36] Although most agree that a heel wedge induces extension of the metacarpophalangeal (MCP) joint, the exact effect remains controversial,[12,29] and it seems that the extension of this joint is associated with lateral axial rotation of the proximal phalanx.[35,37] Furthermore, a strong association exists between loadings of the DIP and MCP joints, and the use of orthopedic shoeing has been shown to affect both joints.[38]

It is generally accepted that heel elevation decreases strain in the DDFT and its accessory ligament, while increasing strain in the SL; however, the effect on the superficial digital flexor tendon remains controversial.[27,38–42] The opposite effects are achieved when a wedge is applied to the toe.[27]

An important effect of elevating the heel is reduction in the force exerted by the DDFT on the navicular bone. A 6° wedge reduces the force by 24%,[12] mainly as a result of reduction in the extending moment arm of the DIP joint but also as a result of the flatter angle of deviation of the tendon around the navicular bone. In a similar way, for every 1° increase in the angle of the distal phalanx to the ground, the force and stress on the navicular bone is calculated to be 6% lower.[13] Heel wedges do not unload the heels,[9] hence it is likely that their use in horses with collapsed heels has to be time limited or the condition may worsen.

THE EFFECT OF APPLYING A SHOE

It is appropriate to evaluate the effect of traditional shoeing on foot biomechanics because, in recent years, the traditional approach of hoof care by farriers and veterinarians has been challenged by various barefoot proponents.[3]

The application of a standard steel shoe to a balanced foot has a minimal effect on the location of the PoF during stance.[9] The weight of a shoe increases inertia; that is, it decreases the ability of the limb to resist changes in velocity of the limb. The weight of the shoe thus creates some changes to variables of the swing phase at high speed,[43–45] and in Icelandic horses during slower toelting speed.[46] Many changes may occur in response to the weight of a shoe, including a slight increase in the loading of a limb, a slightly quicker rotation of the hoof segment, a less vertical hoof lifting,[2] and an increase in the force exerted on the navicular bone by the DDFT by as much as 14%.[12]

Shoeing also alters the concussion-dampening mechanism of the distal limb,[47,48] resulting in increase in the impact on the hoof.[2,49] However, this increase in impact does not seem to extend to the upper limb, because it is largely attenuated at the interface between the hoof wall and distal phalanx. At the level of the MCP joint, the difference between shod and unshod conditions is minimal.[49]

The duration and distance a horse's foot slides after impact is not significantly affected by shoes made of different material,[50] suggesting that horses may have to alter their gait to compensate for the grip characteristics of the shoe, to maintain a constant slip time and distance.[50]

Deceleration force (the rate at which the force decreases at impact) is not significantly different when steel shoes are compared with the unshod condition, but it is significantly smaller with polyurethane shoes,[51] and it is suggested that shoes constructed of compliant materials may mitigate clinical lameness.[51]

Shoeing also elevates the hoof from the ground surface by supporting the hoof wall. This elevation results in less expansion of the palmar aspect of the hoof wall, compared with the unshod horse, although the heel still expands even without contact of the frog with the ground.[52] Shoeing also attenuates contraction of the wall at the heel during the late stages of stance phase.[52] Glued aluminum shoes restrict heel movement even further, potentially interfering with shock absorption.[53] Without a shoe, hoof wall compression at the toe and quarter remains more constant and lower in magnitude than with a shoe. Furthermore, at low weight-bearing loads, shoeing places increased pressure on the frog, which decreases total hoof wall weight bearing and causes palmar movement of the distal phalanx.[54]

However, the significance of the effects described earlier on the hoof, the clinical relevance of the effects of certain shoes, and the relationship of these effects to long-term hoof health is not yet completely understood.

SUMMARY

Fine analysis of the distal limb seems to be limited by the complex anatomy. High-resolution finite element models, generated with data derived from advanced imaging modalities,[55] could give new insight into the biomechanics of the digit, providing new data, unobtainable by other means, for smaller structures of the digit such as the distal sesamoidean, impar, or the collateral ligaments.

Despite the abundance of new information related to the various effects of common shoeing and farriery techniques on foot and lower limb biomechanics, some aspects remain controversial or unclear. A major contributing factor to this is that most studies that have been performed to evaluate the biomechanical effects of shoeing and farriery techniques have been performed using sound horses, and many others have been in vitro studies. Thus, although the information obtained from such studies is interesting, its direct clinical relevance is speculative.

There is still a significant deficit in veterinary knowledge regarding the effects of shoeing and farriery techniques on clinically affected lame horses, or horses with identified clinical conditions, and comparisons of unshod and shod horses are rare. It is hoped that future studies will be performed to bridge this gap, comparing clinically lame horses with sound ones as controls, and/or in prospective designs assessing the long-term effects of any particular technique.

REFERENCES

1. Davies HM. Biomechanics of the equine foot. In: Floyd AE, Mansmann RA, editors. Equine podiatry. St Louis (MO): Saunders Elsevier; 2007. p. 42–56.
2. Roepstorff L, Johnston C, Drevemo S. The effect of shoeing on kinetics and kinematics during the stance phase. Equine Vet J Suppl 1999;30:279–85.

3. Balch OK. Discipline-specific hoof preparation and shoeing. In: Floyd AE, Mansmann RA, editors. Equine podiatry. St Louis (MO): Saunders Elsevier; 2007. p. 393–413.

4. Eliashar E. An evidence-based assessment of the biomechanical effects of the common shoeing and farriery techniques. Vet Clin North Am Equine Pract 2007; 23:425–42.

5. Weishaupt MA, Hogg HP, Auer JA, et al. Velocity-dependent changes of time, force and spatial parameters in Warmblood horses walking and trotting on a treadmill. Equine Vet J Suppl 2010;42:530–7.

6. Crevier-Denoix N, Robin D, Pourcelot P, et al. Ground reaction force and kinematic analysis of limb loading on two different beach sand tracks in harness trotters. Equine Vet J Suppl 2010;42:544–51.

7. Pratt GW. Model for injury to the foreleg of the thoroughbred racehorse. Equine Vet J Suppl 1997;23:30–2.

8. Nigg BM, Herzog W. Biomechanics of the musculoskeletal system. Chichester (England): John Wiley; 1994.

9. Wilson AM, Seelig TJ, Shield RA, et al. The effect of foot imbalance on point of force application in the horse. Equine Vet J 1998;30:540–5.

10. Bartel DL, Schryver HF, Lowe JE, et al. Locomotion in the horse: a procedure for computing the internal forces in the digit. Am J Vet Res 1978;39:1721–7.

11. Eliashar E, McGuigan MP, Rogers KA, et al. A comparison of three horseshoeing styles on the kinetics of breakover in sound horses. Equine Vet J 2002;34:184–90.

12. Willemen MA, Savelberg HH, Barneveld A. The effect of orthopaedic shoeing on the force exerted by the deep digital flexor tendon on the navicular bone in horses. Equine Vet J 1999;31:25–30.

13. Eliashar E, McGuigan MP, Wilson AM. Relationship of foot conformation and force applied to the navicular bone of sound horses at the trot. Equine Vet J 2004;36: 431–5.

14. Wilson AM, McGuigan MP, Fouracre L, et al. The force and contact stress on the navicular bone during trot locomotion in sound horses and horses with navicular disease. Equine Vet J 2001;33:159–65.

15. Clayton HM, Sigafoos R, Curle RD. Effect of three shoe types on the duration of breakover in sound trotting horses. J Equine Vet Sci 1991;11:129–32.

16. Parks A. Form and function of the equine digit. Vet Clin North Am Equine Pract 2003;19:285–308.

17. Hood DM, Taylor D, Wagner IP. Effects of ground surface deformability, trimming, and shoeing on quasistatic hoof loading patterns in horses. Am J Vet Res 2001; 62:895–900.

18. Parks AH. Foot balance, conformation, and lameness. In: Ross MW, Dyson SJ, editors. Diagnosis and management of lameness in the horse. St Louis (MO): Saunders; 2003. p. 250–61.

19. Johnston C, Back W. Hoof ground interaction: when biomechanical stimuli challenge the tissues of the distal limb. Equine Vet J 2006;38:634–41.

20. Ovnicek G, Erfle JB. Wild horse hoof patterns offer a formula for preventing and treating lameness. Proc Am Assoc Equine Pract 1995;41:258–60.

21. van Heel MC, Barneveld A, van Weeren PR, et al. Dynamic pressure measurements for the detailed study of hoof balance: the effect of trimming. Equine Vet J 2004;36:778–82.

22. Moleman M, van Heel MC, van Weeren PR, et al. Hoof growth between two shoeing sessions leads to a substantial increase of the moment about the distal, but not the proximal, interphalangeal joint. Equine Vet J 2006;38:170–4.

23. van Heel MC, van Weeren PR, Back W. Compensation for changes in hoof conformation between shoeing sessions through the adaptation of angular kinematics of the distal segments of the limbs of horses. Am J Vet Res 2006;67: 1199–203.

24. Wright IM, Douglas J. Biomechanical considerations in the treatment of navicular disease. Vet Rec 1993;133:109–14.

25. Wright IM. A study of 118 cases of navicular disease: clinical features. Equine Vet J 1993;25:488–92.

26. Østblom LC, Lund C, Melsen F. Navicular bone disease: results of treatment using egg-bar shoeing technique. Equine Vet J 1984;16:203–6.

27. Riemersma DJ, van den Bogert AJ, Jansen MO, et al. Influence of shoeing on ground reaction forces and tendon strains in the forelimbs of ponies. Equine Vet J 1996;28:126–32.

28. Chateau H, Degueurce C, Denoix JM. Three-dimensional kinematics of the distal forelimb in horses trotting on a treadmill and effects of elevation of heel and toe. Equine Vet J 2006;38:164–9.

29. Scheffer CJ, Back W. Effects of 'navicular' shoeing on equine distal forelimb kinematics on different track surface. Vet Q 2001;23:191–5.

30. Wilson AM, McGuigan MP, Pardoe C. The biomechanical effects of wedged, egg-bar and extension shoes in sound and lame horses. Proc Am Assoc Equine Pract 2001;47:339–43.

31. Clayton HM. Comparison of the stride of trotting horses trimmed with a normal and a broken-back hoof axis. Proc Am Assn Equine Pract 1987;33:289–98.

32. Clayton HM. The effect of an acute hoof wall angulation on the stride kinematics of trotting horses. Equine Vet J Suppl 1990;(9):86–90.

33. Willemen MA, Savelberg HH, Jacobs MW, et al. Biomechanical effects of rocker-toed shoes in sound horses. Vet Q 1996;18(Suppl 2):S75–8.

34. van Heel MC, van Weeren PR, Back W. Shoeing sound Warmblood horses with a rolled toe optimises hoof-unrollment and lowers peak loading during breakover. Equine Vet J 2006;38:258–62.

35. Chateau H, Degueurce C, Denoix JM. Effects of 6 degree elevation of the heels on 3D kinematics of the distal portion of the forelimb in the walking horse. Equine Vet J 2004;36:649–54.

36. Viitanen M, Bird J, Smith R, et al. Biochemical characterisation of navicular hyaline cartilage, navicular fibrocartilage and the deep digital flexor tendon in horses with navicular disease. Res Vet Sci 2003;75:113–20.

37. Chateau H, Degueurce C, Jerbi H, et al. Normal three-dimensional behaviour of the metacarpophalangeal joint and the effect of uneven foot bearing. Equine Vet J Suppl 2001;(33):84–8.

38. Noble P, Lejeune JP, Caudron I, et al. Heel effects on joint contact force components in the equine digit: a sensitivity analysis. Equine Vet J Suppl 2010;42: 475–81.

39. Nilsson G, Fredrickson I, Drevemo S. Some procedures and tools in the diagnostics of distal equine lameness. Acta Vet Scand Suppl 1973;44:63.

40. Lochner FK, Milne DW, Mills EJ, et al. In vivo and in vitro measurement of tendon strain in the horse. Am J Vet Res 1980;41(12):1929–37.

41. Thompson KN, Cheung TK, Silverman BS. The effect of toe angle on tendon, ligament and hoof wall strains in vitro. J Equine Vet Sci 1993;13(11):651–4.

42. Stephens PR, Nunamaker DM, Butterweck DM. Application of a Hall-effect transducer for measurement of tendon strains in horses. Am J Vet Res 1989;50: 1089–95.

43. Willemen MA, Savelberg HH, Bruin G, et al. The effect of toe weights on linear and temporal stride characteristics of standardbred trotters. Vet Q 1994; 16(Supp 2):S97–100.

44. Singelton WH, Clayton HM, Lanovaz JL, et al. Effects of shoeing on forelimb phase kinetics of trotting horses. Vet Comp Orthop Traumatol 2003;16:16–20.

45. Willemen MA, Savelberg HH, Barneveld A. The improvement of the gait quality of sound trotting horses by normal shoeing and its effect on the load of the lower limb. Livest Prod Sci 1998;52:145–53.

46. Rumpler B, Riha A, Licka T, et al. Influence of shoes with different weights on the motion of the limbs in Icelandic horses during toelt at different speeds. Equine Vet J Suppl 2010;42:451–4.

47. Benoit P, Barrey E, Regnault JC, et al. Comparison of the damping effect of different shoeing by the measurement of hoof acceleration. Acta Anat 1993; 146:109–13.

48. Dyhre-Poulsen P, Smedegaard HH, Roed J, et al. Equine hoof function investigated by pressure transducers inside the hoof and accelerometers mounted on the first phalanx. Equine Vet J 1994;26:326–66.

49. Willemen MA, Jacobs MW, Schamhardt HC. In vitro transmission and attenuation of impact vibrations in the distal forelimb. Equine Vet J Suppl 1999;30:245–8.

50. Pardoe CH, McGuigan MP, Rogers KM, et al. The effect of shoe material on the kinetics and kinematics of foot slip at impact on concrete. Equine Vet J Suppl 2001;(33):70–3.

51. Back W, van Schiea MH, Pola JN. Synthetic shoes attenuate hoof impact in the trotting Warmblood horse. Equine Comp Exerc Physiol 2006;3:143–51.

52. Roepstorff L, Johnston C, Drevemo S. In vivo and in vitro heel expansion in relation to shoeing and frog pressure. Equine Vet J Suppl 2001;(33):54–7.

53. Yoshihara E, Takahashi T, Otsuka N, et al. Heel movement in horses: comparison between glued and nailed horse shoes at different speeds. Equine Vet J Suppl 2010;42:431–5.

54. Olivier A, Wannenburg J, Gottschalk RD, et al. The effect of frog pressure and downward vertical load on hoof wall weight-bearing and third phalanx displacement in the horse–an in vitro study. J S Afr Vet Assoc 2001;72:217–27.

55. Collins SN, Murray RC, Kneissl S, et al. Thirty-two component finite element models of a horse and donkey digit. Equine Vet J 2009;41:219–24.

Equine Imaging
The Framework for Applying Therapeutic Farriery

Randy B. Eggleston, DVM

KEYWORDS

- Equine • Therapeutic farriery • Imaging • Radiographs • Lameness

KEY POINTS

- Radiographic evaluation of a horse's foot gives tremendous insight into the relationship between the structures within the foot and between the foot and distal limb.
- The information gained from a radiographic study is highly dependent on the quality of the radiographs.
- A systematic approach should be taken when planning a radiographic study of the foot.
- Taking the time to examine the foot and prepare it properly will avoid the need, risk, and expense of repeating images and will improve the quality and therefore the interpretation of your radiographic images.
- When evaluating the foot for podiatry reasons it is crucial that the positioning of the patient, foot and x-ray beam be flawless.

INTRODUCTION

In equine practice the foot is one of, if not, the most common areas of interest for radiographic evaluation. This radiographic popularity is not only due to the foot being the most common source of lameness but also to the multitude of other indications for radiographic evaluation of the foot. In the absence of lameness, detailed radiographic evaluation of the horse's foot is very useful in guiding the veterinarian and farrier in the prevention of lameness. A horse that exhibits poor foot conformation, imbalance, or abnormal patterns of growth can be a clue to impending foot disease and lameness. Radiographic evaluation of a horse's foot gives tremendous insight into the relationship between the structures within the foot and between the foot and distal limb. When evaluating a horse for purchase, the recommendation for radiographic evaluation of the feet is important in identifying not only previous and existing disease but also the potential for impending foot problems. An underutilized indication for

The author has nothing to disclose.
Large Animal Surgery, Department of Large Animal Medicine, College of Veterinary Medicine, University of Georgia, 501 DW Brooks Drive, Athens, GA 30602, USA
E-mail address: egglesto@uga.edu

radiographic evaluation of the foot is in consultation with the farrier. A relationship between the veterinarian and farrier must be present to maintain and preserve the health of the horse's foot and to incorporate the skills and knowledge of the farrier to formulate solutions for the problem foot. It is the combination of the medical and surgical expertise of the veterinarian and the skills and expertise of the farrier that results in a successful outcome for the horse and owner. It is also through this relationship that the veterinarian gains an appreciation for the skills and knowledge of the farrier (ie, types of shoes and their purpose) as well as the farrier gaining an appreciation for the knowledge and expertise of the veterinarian (ie, radiographic interpretation of the foot).

The information gained from a radiographic study is highly dependent on the quality of the radiographs ("garbage in, garbage out"). It is imperative that the veterinarian invest in quality equipment, become proficient at operating the equipment, and make the effort to set up technique charts, with the goal of producing consistent and quality radiographic studies. Radiographic evaluation of the horse's foot does not replace the need for a detailed physical examination and lameness evaluation, including diagnostic anesthesia. A systematic approach should be taken when planning a radiographic study of the foot; the "point and shoot" approach is not always the best approach. Taking multiple standard views, although not always necessary, is important to help avoid a missed diagnosis. Frequently, additional projections may be required to further investigate initial findings or confirm a diagnosis. There are a number of preplanning questions that need to be asked before performing foot radiographs: What is the purpose of the study (investigation of lameness or consultation with the farrier)? What do I expect to gain from the study (source of lameness or information useful in managing the foot)? What information do I need to obtain from the study (relationship of the hoof capsule and the distal phalanx)? The answers to these questions will guide in planning the study with regard to the appropriate views to be taken, the appropriate technique, and the appropriate positioning of the foot and centering of the x-ray beam.

EQUIPMENT

Digital radiography (DR) is now commonplace in equine practice. Although expensive, the advantages over film/screen radiography and the demand for digital radiography make it a worthwhile investment. The advantages of DR over film/screen radiography include improved image quality, digital postprocessing, and improved archiving. Digital radiographs have tremendous exposure latitude compared with plain film radiography, which results in far fewer retakes and reduced radiation exposure to personnel. With a single image from a single exposure, the clinician has the ability to adjust brightness and contrast to improve detection of subtle lesions or those at the extremes of optical density. Once captured, processed, and saved, the images can be archived electronically, eliminating the need for film storage. The ability to transmit the images quickly for the purpose of consultation, second opinions, and prepurchase examinations allows the practitioner to practice more efficiently and better serve the client.[1] DR has allowed identification and more accurate diagnosis of some lesions in the foot that were otherwise difficult to visualize or questionable at best. It has also introduced questions about the significance of observations that were not previously visible.[2]

Once obtained, digital radiographs can be viewed and manipulated by a number of different software packages or picture archiving and communication systems (PACS). Software viewers provide the user with tools to manipulate the image such as contrast, brightness, magnification, color inversion, etc, as well as the ability to measure angles and distances, rotate, flip, annotate, and save images in standard graphic-file formats (jpeg, tiff, or bmp).[1] Despite the advantages of digital technology, like any imaging technology, it has its limitations. Furthermore, high-quality conventional radiographs are satisfactorily diagnostic for many purposes. However, because there is less exposure latitude with conventional film/screen radiography, when there is a high range of radiographic densities, it is important to establish standard technique charts, taking into consideration the view to be taken, what information is to be obtained from the particular view, and the size of the foot. Additionally, because the same degree of detail and contrast are not as obvious on conventional film, establishing multiple techniques (soft tissue and bone) for each view is necessary to visualize and evaluate soft and osseous tissues.[3]

Additional equipment required to obtain quality radiographs include positioning blocks and appropriate markers. There are commercial positioning blocks and stands available for equine practice that aid in standardizing focal distance, foot placement, and alignment of the x-ray beam. Wood blocks of the appropriate size and height work well; commercial blocks are available but they are also simple to fabricate to the practitioner's desired specifications. A variation to the standard flat block is one that the author uses and is composed of 2 independent circular blocks connected in such a way that allows rotation of the 2 halves (**Fig. 1**). A copper wire is embedded in the surface of the block, forming a 15-cm circle; this acts as a radiographic marker for the weight-bearing surface. Radiographically, regardless of the beam angle with the surface of the block, a line drawn from the 2 apices of the ellipse will be parallel to the weight bearing surface. This block is based on one originally described by Caudron and colleagues.[4] This works well for horses that exhibit conformational faults such as a toed-in or toed-out conformation. When the foot is placed on the block, the rotation of the block allows the foot to position itself naturally, influenced by the horse's conformation, and thereby alleviating the possibility of positional artifacts such as joint space asymmetry. When designing or purchasing a positioning block, it is important to take into consideration the height of the block and the x-ray machine used. Proper positioning will be discussed in later sections. Incorporating some type of metallic marker within the surface of the block is useful in aiding accurate identification of the ground surface, thus improving the accuracy of foot measurements.

Using the appropriate markers and following the standards for marker placement are important in identifying the appropriate foot and orientation of the x-ray beam.[5]

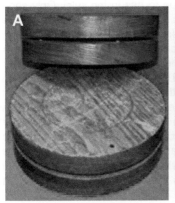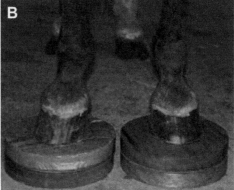

Fig. 1. Rotating positioning block. (*A*) Note copper metal insert used for identification of weight-bearing surface. (*B*) Rotation of the block allows for accurate placement of the limb due to variations in conformation.

This is particularly important when comparing archived images for the purpose of monitoring the response to a trimming or shoeing prescription.

- Marker is placed either lateral or dorsal to the area of interest.
- Lateral marker placement takes precedence over dorsal marker placement.
- On a dorsal-lateral-palmar-medial-oblique view, the marker will project on the palmar side of the foot.
- On a dorsal-medial-palmar-lateral-oblique view, the marker will project on the dorsal side of the foot.

PREPARATION AND POSITIONING OF THE FOOT

Taking the time to examine the foot and prepare it properly will avoid the need, risk, and expense of repeating images and will improve the quality and therefore the interpretation of your radiographic images. It is usual to recommend removing the shoes before performing a full series of foot radiographs. However, depending on the information needed from a study, the radiographs can frequently be taken with the shoes in place. For example, performing radiographs with the shoes in place can be useful when consulting with the farrier. Being able to visualize the shoe allows the clinician to accurately identify the weight-bearing surface and the position of the shoe in relation to the hoof capsule and distal phalanx. This simplifies evaluation of the point of breakover, sole depth and balance of the foot. If a source of lameness has been localized to the foot, removal of the shoes may be needed to obtain the additional views necessary to fully evaluate the foot. Acquiring owner permission to remove shoes is often overlooked but is important for client relations. Proper shoe removal technique is a skill with which the veterinarian must be comfortable. An owner may request that their farrier or the veterinarian may request that the owner's farrier prepare the foot before performing a radiographic study.

The foot should be thoroughly cleansed with a stiff brush, and soap and water if necessary. Once the gross debris is removed, the outer wall and the sole should be evaluated for any frog overgrowth or flaky sole that must be removed to reduce the potential for gas artifact. Any flakiness or accumulations on the outer wall can be removed with either a rasp or a sanding block. Once the foot is prepared, packing the sulci (using Play-Doh [Hasbro, Pawtucket, RI, USA] or appropriate putty material) reduces the likelihood of radiographic artifact due to gas in the sulci. Only enough packing material should be used to fill the depths of the sulci; overpacking will cause packing artifact along the margins of the packing. In horses that have deep center sulci or overgrown bars, alleviation of all gas artifacts can be difficult with routine packing. Placing the foot in a water bath is an effective method of displacing trapped gas to eliminate gas shadows from the image (**Fig. 2**). The vessel that is used should have a flat bottom, preferably without molded supporting ridges. The water depth should be at a level just proximal to the heel bulbs. Keeping the level to a minimum will help reduce the reluctance of the horse to keep the foot placed and reduce radiographic scatter. It is also recommended that the cassette or digital sensor be placed in a plastic protective cover (trash bag) prior to placement of the foot. A 50% increase in technique is recommended when using DR; when using film-screen radiography, a significant increase in milliamperage seconds (mAs) will also be necessary and will depend on whether a grid is used (**Fig. 3**).

When evaluating a foot's conformation and balance, accurately identifying points (land marks) on the foot aid in evaluating the dorsal hoof wall and heel angles, sole depth, and medial and lateral wall height. Although DR allows improved visualization

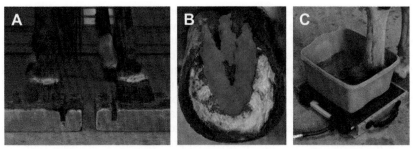

Fig. 2. Foot preparation for radiographic study. (*A*) Right front foot has been properly prepared for imaging. (*B*) Bottom of the foot has been packed with Play-Doh (Hasbro), which displaces trapped gas and alleviates gas artifact on radiographic image. (*C*) Foot is placed in a water bath, resulting in displacement of gas in areas that traditional packing sometimes fails to displace.

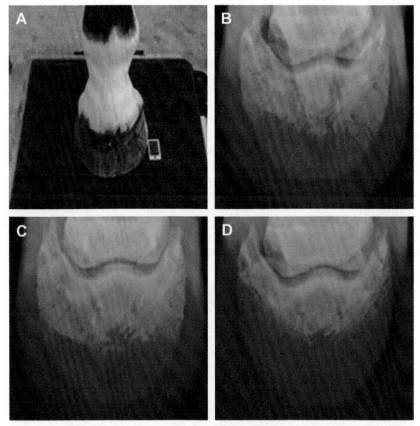

Fig. 3. (*A*) DP-45-PDO. (*B*) Radiographic image of a foot that has not been packed. Note the artifact associated with the sulci of the foot. (*C*) Traditional packing with Play-Doh (Hasbro) alleviates the majority of artifacts; however, packing artifact can still be present. (*D*) Foot is placed in a water bath, resulting in displacement of all gas and packing artifacts.

of soft tissues, accurate identification of the coronary band and heels can be difficult. Rigid metallic markers are often used to identify the true border of the dorsal wall; however, accurate identification of the wall length is often difficult, particularly at the heels. Running a 2-mm bead of barium paste (can be easily stored in and applied from a 60-mL syringe) directly over the dorsal median hoof wall extending from the coronary band to the tip of the toe allows for accurate identification of the wall border, toe length, and appreciation of hoof wall distortion. Placing a small dollop of paste at the following points will aid in the evaluation of quarter angles, quarter wall height, heel angle and height, sole depth, and toe-to-heel ratio: (1) widest point of the proximal (coronary) and distal wall in the quarters, (2) proximal and distal wall in the heels, and (3) at the apex of the frog (**Fig. 4**).

When evaluating the foot for podiatry reasons, it is crucial that the positioning of the patient, foot, and x-ray beam be flawless. Accurate assessment and measurement of the dorsal hoof wall and heel angle, sole depth, joint congruity, medial-to-lateral (M-L) balance, and toe-to-heel ratio are dependent on proper positioning.

The horse should be placed on a firm level footing with the limbs squarely beneath them. Slight abduction or adduction of the limb or shifting of weight can cause joint incongruity on the horizontal beam dorsopalmar view (HD-P) (**Fig. 5**). When placing the foot on the positioning blocks, it is also important to allow the foot to position itself as dictated by the limb conformation (toed-in, toed-out); this is where the rotating blocks are helpful. Having a level, consistent surface also allows more accurate alignment of the x-ray machine for the lateromedial (L-M) and HD-P/plantar projections. To reduce magnification, the foot should be placed on the positioning block in such a way the foot makes contact with the cassette or sensor plate.

X-RAY BEAM ORIENTATION

Focal-film distance should be kept constant for all projections. Changes in the focal-film distance will alter the exposure of the image assuming the exposure settings are held constant.

Distortion of the radiographic image occurs if the x-ray beam is not perpendicular to the radiographic cassette or sensor unit. Distortion to the horizontal projections (L-M, HD-P/plantar) will result in asymmetry within the image and inaccurate evaluation of the image and radiographic measurements. Magnification increases as the distance from the cassette or sensor unit to the object increases or when the distance from the focal spot to the object decreases. This can be minimized with proper placement

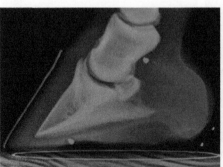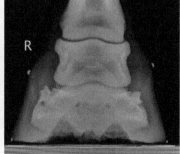

Fig. 4. Radiopaque markers placed at the appropriate locations aides in accurate identification of coronary band and distal hoof wall.

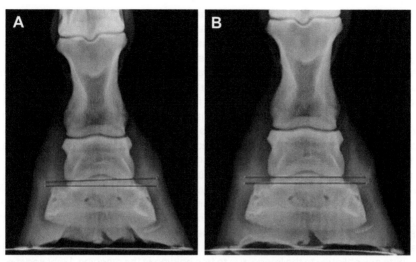

Fig. 5. HD-P projection showing abnormal and normal DIP joint symmetry in the same horse. (A) The limb is slightly abducted and the horses weight is shifted to the contralateral limb. (B) The horse is positioned squarely with both front limbs directly underneath him and standing on identical positioning blocks.

of the foot on the positioning blocks. There is more image distortion of the dorsopalmar/plantar radiograph due to the angle of the pastern, but placing the cassette parallel with the pastern will create distortion of the foot, which is unacceptable. Therefore, the slight magnification produced with this view is acceptable and does not make a significant change to the interpretation of the image.[3] A plantar/palmarodorsal projection can be taken to reduce magnification, but it is not necessary and can be unsafe to personnel and equipment.

In positioning the x-ray beam, consideration of the area of interest as well as a good understanding of foot anatomy is important. Beam angle is most important in the L-M and dorsopalmar/plantar projections. For example, in the L-M projection the beam should be aligned parallel with the heel bulbs. In the majority of feet, this will produce a lateral image resulting in superimposition of the palmar/plantar eminences of the distal phalanx and an absence of horizontal obliquity to the distal interphalangeal (DIP) joint (**Fig. 6**). In the HD-P projection, the alignment of the beam should be in the sagittal plane

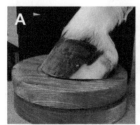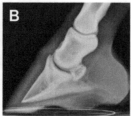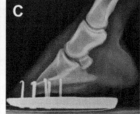

Fig. 6. L-M projection. (A, B) The beam orientation is perpendicular to the dorsopalmar plane of the foot. Parallel alignment with the heel bulbs is useful in proper alignment of the x-ray machine. The beam is centered at a point half way between the toe and the heels and 1.5 to 2 cm proximal to the weight-bearing surface. (C) Shoe placement and point of breakover can be evaluated with L-M projection taken with the shoe on.

and at an angle perpendicular to a line parallel to the heel bulbs. When viewing the image, the apex of the extensor process of the distal phalanx should be projected on the mid-sagittal plane of the second phalanx, indicating a true dorsopalmar image **(Fig. 7)**. The beam should always be parallel with the ground surface. In addition to beam angle, proper aiming of the central beam is required and is dictated by the type of study being performed and the specific area of interest. If the area of interest is the distal phalanx and the purpose of the study is evaluating foot balance and symmetry, the center of the beam on the L-M projection should be aimed 1.5 to 2.0 cm proximal to the weight-bearing surface and midway between the toe and the heel (see **Fig. 6**). The goal of this image is to have the medial and lateral solar margins of the distal phalanx superimposed on one another. If there is obliquity in the image, 1 of 2 things need to be considered: the x-ray beam needs to be adjusted based on the sole depth of the foot, or the beam orientation is correct for that foot but the horse is exhibiting some degree of M-L imbalance or poor hoof conformation causing obliquity of the foot itself; this can later be confirmed on the HD-P/plantar projection **(Fig. 8)**. Depending on the height of the positioning block, height adjustments can be easily made by placing the machine on spacers of the appropriate thickness to bring the beam to the desired height. This helps eliminate any obliquity to the image due to free holding of the machine. Light sedation is often necessary and can help maintain positioning through the study. Regardless of whether a unilateral or bilateral study is being performed, both feet should be placed on blocks of equal height. Correct positioning reduces the likelihood of artifactual changes to the joint space that might otherwise be interpreted as joint asymmetry and foot imbalance (see **Fig. 5**).

EXPOSURE

In addition to foot preparation, limb positioning and beam orientation, proper exposure settings (kVp and mAs) are important in obtaining the optimal image. To fully evaluate the foot, multiple plain film images taken at different exposures are needed to appreciate changes to different tissues of the foot (soft tissue and bone). This again is one of the major advantages of digital radiography over film/screen radiography. Exposure latitude with DR is substantially greater than that of conventional film/screen

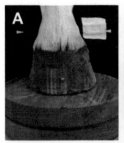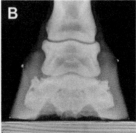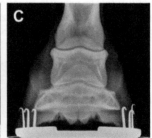

Fig. 7. HD-P projection. (*A*) The beam orientation is parallel to the dorsopalmar plane of the foot and bisecting the axial plane of the foot. As with the L-M projection, the x-ray beam is targeted 1.5 to 2 cm above the weight-bearing surface of the foot or 7 cm distal to the dorsal coronary band on a line perpendicular to the weight-bearing surface. (*B*) Placement of a radiopaque marker on the axial-dorsal surface of the wall helps in accurate identification of the extent of the hoof capsule. (*C*) Shoe placement and accurate assessment of distal medial and lateral aspect of the wall can be evaluated with L-M projection taken with the shoe on.

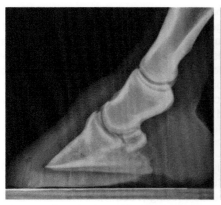
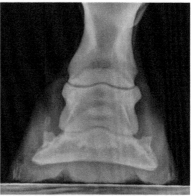

Fig. 8. Lateral projection with proper alignment of the x-ray beam demonstrating uneven alignment of the solar margins of the distal phalanx in a horse with poor conformation. Evaluation of the HD-P projection confirms the presence of poor hoof conformation.

radiography.[1] Although the exposure range is larger for DR, using proper exposure settings is important to reduce underexposure and overexposure of the initial image.[1,6] Once the image is obtained, computer manipulation (brightness and contrast) of that image allows enhancement of the soft tissue and bone densities within the foot from a single exposure. With film/screen radiography, multiple images taken at different exposures are necessary to enhance the soft tissue and bony structures of the foot.

An underexposed digital radiograph occurs when too few x-rays are detected by the imaging plate and will result in a grainy, noisy, mottled, and pixilated appearance and a decrease in image quality. Increasing exposure settings will remedy this artifact. An overexposed digital radiograph can result in multiple artifacts. Moderate overexposure will result in an image that is light, white, or pale.[6–8] As the exposure increases, areas of minimal x-ray attenuation, such as the periphery of a structure, will be obliterated due to oversaturation of the detector system and that portion of the image is no longer viewable.[7,8] Another common overexposure artifact that is seen is rectangular areas of differing intensity throughout the background of the image; this is referred to as "planking."[7,8] Reducing exposure settings will generally alleviate all of these overexposure artifacts (**Fig. 9**). Computer manipulation of an image that is underexposed

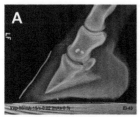
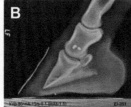
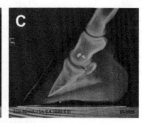

Fig. 9. Images depiciting normal and abnormal exposure settings and the artifacts produced by those exposures. (*A*) Underexposed image; note the low exposure index (EI) (43) and the grainy pixilated appearance of the image. (*B*) Proper exposure setting; note the EI of 251. (*C*) Overexposed image; note the high EI of 1038 and the planking and loss of soft tissue margins in the image.

or overexposed will not produce an image that is comparable to one taken with optimal technique.[7] When a digital image is generated, a figure is displayed that is referred to as the exposure index, S value, REX No., DDI, or IgM value. This value is an estimation of whether an exposure is appropriate based on the manufacturer's recommendations for that particular system.[6,8] This value should be used as a guideline to determine if an image should be repeated or if computer manipulation is adequate. To minimize exposure artifacts, technique charts should be used with settings specific for tissue thickness and the region of interest.

VIEWS

The 2 radiographic views most commonly used for farriery are the L-M and the HD-P views. In the presence of lameness, multiple other views are needed and can also be useful to the farrier in prescribing therapeutic shoeing (**Table 1**).

L-M View

The L-M view is performed with the horse standing squarely on a flat level surface with each foot on a position block of equal height; when standing in this manner the metacarpus/metatarsus of a horse without an angular deformity at the carpus should be vertical. Focal-film distance usually ranges between 24 and 28 inches and will vary with the specific film-screen combination and technique chart that is developed. It is important to be consistent and, once the technique is established, the focal-film distance should remain constant. The beam is centered at a point midway between the toe and the heels and 1.5 to 2 cm proximal to the weight-bearing surface (see **Fig. 6**).[3,9] This beam alignment will produce a film that shows the medial and lateral solar margins and palmar processes of the distal phalanx superimposed on one another (in the "normal" foot) allowing for accurate evaluation of the dorsopalmar balance of the foot. This projection is useful in evaluating location of the breakover, shoe placement, and quantitatively evaluating the foot. Useful parameters that should be obtained include the dorsal hoof wall length (DHWL), angle (DHWA), and wall thickness (DHT), the distance between the dorsal coronary band and the apex of the extensor process (CED), also referred to as the founder distance, the angle between the solar margin of the distal phalanx and the ground surface, also referred to as solar

Table 1
Recommended radiographic views of the foot based on desired study

Study	Projection
Foot balance	L-M
Podiatry	HD-P
Farrier consultation	
Laminitis	
Lameness/prepurchase examination	L-M
	HD-P
	DP-45-PDO
	DP-60-PDO
	PP-PDO
Additional views	DLP-45-PMDO
	DMP-45-PLDO
	Horizontal dorsolateral–(45°)–palmaromedial oblique (HDL-45-PMO)
	Horizontal dorsomedial–(45°)–palmarolateral oblique (HDM-45-PLO)

or palmar angle (SA), the sole depth (SD), the angle of the heel (HA), and the distribution of the dorsal and palmar portions of the foot, separated by a line extending from the center of rotation of the DIP joint, perpendicular to the weight-bearing surface, referred to as the toe:foot ratio (T:F). If the navicular bone is the prime area of interest, the x-ray beam should be centered at a point halfway between the dorsal and palmar coronary band, and approximately 1 cm distal to the coronary band. For the DIP joint, the x-ray beam is centered on the coronary band at the junction of the dorsal and middle third of the coronary band (**Fig. 10**).

Interpretation

Once the image is acquired, what useful information can be obtained? This view is useful in evaluating the relationship of the distal phalanx with the hoof capsule as well as with the distal limb (hoof-pastern axis). Malalignment of the foot and pastern is seen in 72.8% of horses with forelimb lameness.[10] Assuming foot placement and beam alignment are consistent, malalignment of the medial and lateral solar margins is indicative of M-L imbalance in the foot or poor conformation and can be confirmed with evaluation of the HD-P (see **Fig. 8**). Resorption and remodeling of the distal phalanx can alter the dorsal contour, solar margins, and length of the distal phalanx as well as alter the shape and angle of the solar margin, complicating interpretation. These changes are seen with laminitis, pedal osteitis, and other sources of chronic inflammation (heel bulb avulsions, osteomyelitis, etc.).

Quantitative methods of evaluating the horse's foot have been developed.[11] These parameters are obtained from L-M and HD-P radiographic images. Changes in or manipulation of these parameters have been used to evaluate, the effects of trimming and shoeing,[10,12,13] the affects of changing hoof angle on the stresses delivered to the deep digital flexor tendon (DDFT),[14,15] the relationship between foot conformation and lameness,[16–18] and the relationship between SA and DDFT injuries in the thoroughbred.[14]

Parameters most useful in evaluating the horses foot include the DHWL, DHWA, DHT, CED, SA, SD, HA, and T:F (**Fig. 11**). Subjective assessment of a well-taken radiograph is frequently adequate for evaluating the horse's foot; quantitative assessment

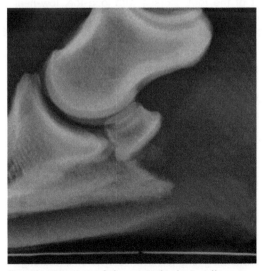

Fig. 10. Properaly aligned projection of the navicular bone allows assesment of the proximal, distal, flexor (palmar), and dorsal boarders as well as the medullary cavity.

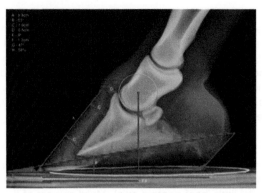

Fig. 11. Measured L-M projection. Quantitative assessment of the horse's foot. (A) DHWL. (B) DHWA. (C, C′) (H-L zone), DHWT. (D) CED. (E) SA. (F) SD. (G) HA. (H) T:F.

is useful in documenting changes in a foot over time and when comparing feet on the same horse.

The L-M projection assesses change in the dorsopalmar balance of the foot as represented by changes in the DHWA, SA, and disproportionate distribution of foot mass in relation to the center of rotation. Minimal decreases or flattening of the SA and DHWA have been associated with lameness.[19] There is a wide range in what is considered normal for the SA (2°–8°).[10–12,14,18–20] In one study, it was concluded that an increase in the solar angle by 1° would decrease the DDFT force, and therefore, its force on the navicular bone, by 4%. The distribution of foot mass is separated by the center of rotation (COR). The COR is located midway between the dorsal and palmar aspects of the distal articular surface of the middle phalanx; a line dropped from this point and perpendicular to the weight-bearing surface divides the dorsal palmar foot mass. The T:F in the normal foot should be between 60% and 67%.[10,21] If viewed from the solar surface of the foot, the COR should correspond to the widest point of the foot. Horses with long-toe, low-heel syndrome tend to have a long narrow frog, low DHWA and SA, and disproportionate distribution of sole mass with excessive mass dorsal to the center of rotation (>67%) (**Fig. 12**). A solar

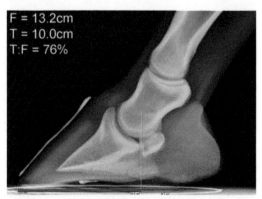

Fig. 12. Image demonstarating long toe/low heel syndrome resulting in an abnormal distribution of sole mass in relation to the COR. Seventy-six percent of the sole mass is dorsal to the COR.

angle of less than 2° is usually associated with a dorsopalmar imbalance; the center of rotation of the DIP joint is displaced toward the heels, resulting in an increase in the T:F ratio.[22]

Trimming and shoeing the horse's foot impact all but 2 of these parameters (DHT, CED) and result in an overall change in the equilibrium and balance of the foot. Repeating the L-M projection following trimming and shoeing the foot is useful in evaluating the affects of the trim.

Additional radiographic abnormalities seen in this projection include changes to the solar margin in horses with pedal osteitis, small focal irregularities at the insertions of the deep digital flexor tendon and the distal sesamoidean impar ligament, and osteophyte or enthesophyte formation associated with the DIP joint. Some clinicians also consider this projection to be sensitive in the identification of navicular disease, as a well-positioned L-M projection focused on the navicular bone allows for evaluation of all borders of the bone and the changes to the medullary cavity (see **Fig. 10**).[9]

HD-P View

This view is also performed with the horse standing squarely on 2 positioning blocks with the foot placed toward the back of the block. The cassette is placed on the palmar surface perpendicular to the floor. The focal-film distance remains constant. The beam orientation is parallel to the dorsopalmar long axis of the foot on the median plane of the foot. As with the L–M projection, the x-ray beam is centered 1.5 to 2 cm above the weight-bearing surface of the foot (**Fig. 13A**). It is this projection where the dynamic rotary block may add additional accuracy to the interpretation of the image, alleviating artifact due to conformation or foot placement. Placement of a small dot of barium paste or an alternative radiopaque marker at the hairline on the medial and lateral coronet may help in accurate identification of the proximal-most extent of the medial and lateral coronet (**Fig. 13B**).

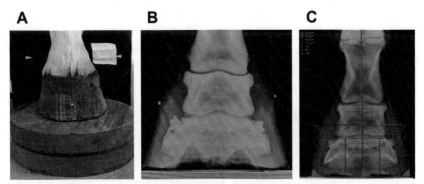

Fig. 13. HD-P projection. (A) The beam orientation is parallel to the dorsopalmar plane of the foot and bisecting the axial plane of the foot. As with the L-M projection, the x-ray beam is targeted 1.5 to 2 cm above the weight-bearing surface of the foot or 7 cm distal to the dorsal coronary band on a line perpendicular to the weight-bearing surface. (B) Placement of a radiopaque marker on the axial-dorsal surface of the wall helps in accurate identification of the extents of the hoof capsule. (C) Measured HD-P projection. Quantitative assessment of the horse's foot. (A) Lateral hoof wall length (LHWL). (B) Medial hoof wall length (MHWL). (C) Lateral distal phalanx height (LP3H). (D) Medial distal phalanx height (MP3H). (E) Lateral hoof wall angle (LHWA). (F) Medial hoof wall angle (MHWA). (G) Median angle (MA).

Interpretation

This projection allows evaluation of M-L balance and conformation of the foot with observation and measurement of the medial and lateral wall length and angle and the orientation of the distal phalanx within the hoof capsule. Orientation of the distal phalanx can be assessed by measuring the distance from the articular surface of the distal phalanx to the ground surface; the solar canal can also be used as a reference point, but it is less consistent. Using the solar margin as a point of reference can be variable due to changes that can occur in the bone. Ideally, the articular surface of the distal phalanx is parallel to the ground as is a line between the medial and lateral coronary band. Additionally, the medial and lateral walls are of equal thickness, and the distances from the medial and lateral solar margins to the ground are the same (see **Fig. 13C**). Furthermore, the DIP joint space should be even across its width. It is normal for the medial quarter wall to be at a slightly steeper angle and subsequently measure shorter in length.[22] Asymmetry in medial and lateral wall length and angle are a common radiographic finding in the D-P image; if the proximal interphalangeal and DIP joint spaces are congruent, the significance of this asymmetry is questionable.[22] Any incongruency in the DIP joint indicates M-L imbalance and should be considered significant (**Fig. 14**).[22] However, caution in overinterpretation of joint incongruency is recommended because any malpositioning of the limb or foot can create the appearance of M-L imbalance. It is important that the cannon bone be perpendicular to the floor in both the M-L and dorsopalmar planes. Keeping the horse's head and neck straight is also important to reduce the influence of uneven loading of any one limb (see **Fig. 5**).

Dorsoproximal–(45°)–Palmarodistal/Plantar Oblique (DP-45-PDO)

The DP-45-PDO view is performed with the horse standing squarely on a positioning tunnel. This projection is also described as being performed in the non–weight-bearing limb with an assortment of different positioning blocks (eg, navicular block).

It is not critical that both feet be placed on similar tunnels. The beam orientation is parallel with the dorsopalmar, median plane of the foot. The beam is also oriented in a dorsoproximal-to-palmarodistal direction, 45° to the weight-bearing surface and the long axis of the limb. The beam is centered 1 cm distal to the coronary band (**Fig. 15**).

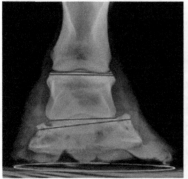 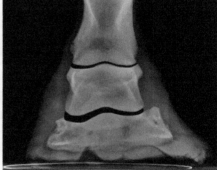

Fig. 14. Severe M-L imbalance causing flaring of the lateral hoof wall. Note the incongruency in the proximal interphalangeal and DIP joint spaces.

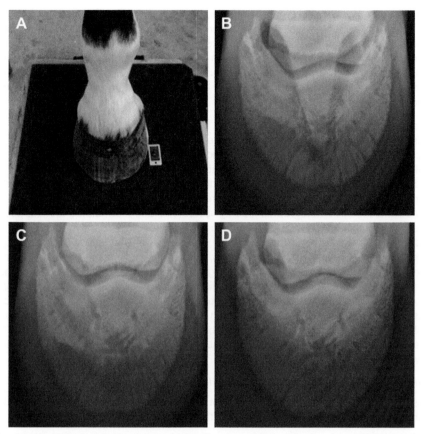

Fig. 15. DP-45-PDO. (*A*) The beam orientation is parallel with the dorsopalmar, sagittal plane of the foot. The beam is aimed in a proximodorsal-to-palmarodistal direction, 45° to the weight-bearing surface and the long axis of the limb. The beam should be centered 1 cm distal to the coronary band. (*B*) Gas artifact is obvious through the sulci of the un-packed foot. (*C*) Traditional packing alleviates the majority of artifacts; however, packing artifact can still be present. (*D*) Use of the water bath displaces all gas and packing artifacts.

Interpretation

This projection allows inspection of the solar border of the distal phalanx. Changes to the solar border of the distal phalanx can vary considerably. Resorption of the solar border can be secondary to aseptic or septic inflammation, or neoplasia. Aseptic oste-itis may present with focal resorption with a smooth rim of sclerosis, whereas septic osteitis will exhibit an irregular moth eaten area with bony sequestration.[9] Osteitis may also cause a widening of the radiating vascular channels. Most distal phalanx fractures are best identified with this projection. Additional potential changes that should be evaluated include sclerosis or lysis at the insertion of the collateral ligaments within the fossae located at the lateral and medial articular margins of the DIP joint, navicular fractures, and changes in the DIP joint space.[9]

Dorsoproximal–600–Palmarodistal/Plantar (DP-60-PDO)

The DP-60-PDO projection is taken with an increased technique compared to the DP-45-PDO projection, also with the horse standing squarely with the foot of interest on a positioning tunnel. The purpose of this projection is evaluation of the navicular bone. Because of the narrow area of interest the beam should be collimated lightly so that it is just enough to cover the navicular bone. The beam orientation is similar to that of the 45° projection except that the beam angle is increased to 60° from the weight-bearing surface or 30° from the long axis of the limb. The beam should be centered at a position 1 cm proximal to the coronary band in the median plane of the foot (**Fig. 16**).

Interpretation

This technique results in penetration of the overlying middle and distal phalanx and improved detail of the proximal, distal, and lateral borders of the navicular bone as well as the medullary cavity. There is debate regarding the normal acceptable shape and size of the navicular bone and its contribution to a diagnosis of navicular disease. Numerous studies have attempted to correlate navicular changes to a diagnosis of navicular disease. A radiographic grading system has been formulated to more accurately and objectively classify these changes and correlate them to clinical lameness.[9,23,24] The changes that correlate strongly with lameness include large medullary lucencies, medullary sclerosis, and bony remodeling at the proximal border.[9,24] Although difficult to identify, fragmentation of the distal border at the junction of the horizontal border and the medial and lateral oblique angles of the bone should be evaluated. Navicular bone fractures are also identified in this projection. Gas artifact from poorly prepared sulci can be mistaken for fracture lines, but artifactual lines will project beyond the margins of the bone. Repacking the foot should be attempted or, as preferred by this author, using a water bath to completely displace any gas artifact.

Palmaroproximal–Palmarodistal Oblique (Flexor Tangential) (PP-PDO)

This projection is performed with the foot placed on a positioning tunnel with the limb of interest positioned palmar to the midstance position. This results in

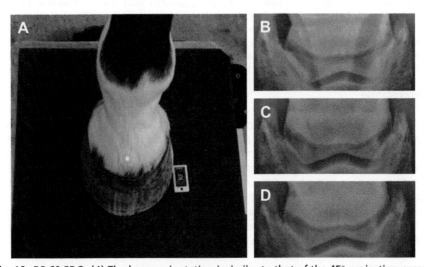

Fig. 16. DP-60-PDO. (*A*) The beam orientation is similar to that of the 45° projection except for the beam angle is increased to 60° from the weight-bearing surface. The beam should be targeted at a position 1 cm proximal to the coronary band in the axial plane of the foot. (*B*) Unpacked. (*C*) Packed with Play-Doh (Hasbro). (*D*) Foot in a water path.

increased dorsiflexion of the DIP joint and the metacarpal phalangeal joint, thereby "opening" the back of the foot and pastern. The focal–film distance is usually limited by the abdomen of the horse. The x-ray beam is oriented in the palmaroproximal-to-palmarodistal angle with the beam following the angle of the palmar surface of the pastern and centered directly in the divot formed between the collateral cartilages (**Fig. 17**).

Interpretation

This projection allows evaluation of the flexor surface, flexor cortex, and axial portion of the medullary cavity of the navicular bone as well as the palmar processes of the distal phalanx. Common radiographic abnormalities of the palmar processes include irregular bony margins consistent with pedal osteitis and fractures. This projection is most useful for evaluation of the navicular bone. The most significant radiographic changes include poor corticomedullary definition, medullary sclerosis, and changes to the contour of the flexor surface.[9,24]

Additional Views

Additional views of the foot are often indicated based on physical examination, lameness examination, and survey films. Horizontal beam oblique projections can be performed to look at the dorsomedial and dorsolateral surfaces of the distal phalanx (**Fig. 18**).[25] The beam orientation is similar to that of the horizontal beam projections except that it is oriented in either a dorsolateral-to-palmaromedial or dorsomedial-to-palmarolateral direction. The lateral borders of the navicular bone and palmar eminences of the distal phalanx can also be more extensively evaluated. Dorsoproximal oblique views allow for more accurate evaluation of the palmar processes and particularly for identification of abaxial distal phalanx fractures. These projections are performed with the horse standing squarely and positioned on positioning tunnels. The x-ray beam is oriented in a dorsolateral proximal–(45°)–palmaromedial distal oblique (DLP-45-PMDO) or dorsomedial proximal–(45°)–palmarolateral distal oblique (DMP-45-PLDO) direction. The beam is centered

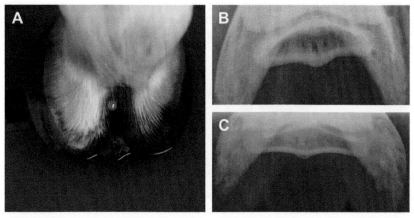

Fig. 17. PP-PDO. (*A*) The x-ray beam is oriented in the palmaroproximal-to-palmarodistal angle with the beam following the angle of the palmar surface of the pastern and centered directly in the divot formed by the heel bulbs. (*B*) Packed with Play-Doh (Hasbro). (*C*) Foot in water bath.

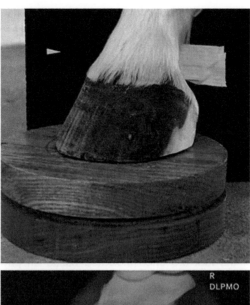

Fig. 18. Horizontal dorsolateral–(45°)–palmaromedial oblique (HDL-45-PMO) projection. The beam orientation is in the horizontal plane 45° dorsolateral or dorsomedial and centered 1.5 to 2 cm proximal to the weight-bearing surface.

on a point just distal to the coronary band and between the lateral quarter and heel. The obliquity of the beam off lateral can be altered, which will allow visualization of different aspects of the DIP articular margins and lateral margins of the navicular bone (**Fig. 19**).

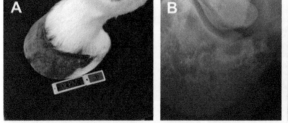
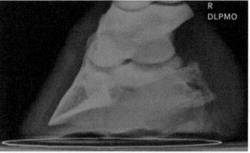
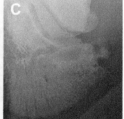

Fig. 19. DLP-45-PMDO projection. (*A*) The x-ray beam is oriented in a DLP-45-PMDO or DMP-45-PLDO direction. The beam is centered on a point just distal to the coronary band and between the lateral quarter and heel. The obliquity of the beam off lateral can be altered, which will allow visualization of different aspects of the DIP articular margins and lateral margins of the navicular bone. (*B*) Packed with Play-Doh (Hasbro). (*C*) Foot in water bath.

SUMMARY

Imaging of the equine foot has made tremendous advancements in the past 10 to 12 years with the introduction of magnetic resonance imaging allowing an understanding of its normal anatomy and how it relates to lameness; however, for the practitioner, radiography of the foot remains the most practical, economical, and informative imaging modality in the field. Having said that, the quality of the information gained from a radiograph is only as good as the quality of the radiograph itself. Using high-quality equipment, maintaining that equipment, and mastering radiographic technique and image acquisition are imperative to obtaining quality information. Depending on the information desired from a radiographic study, a limited number of views are required. Based on the information gained from the standard study and the clinical presentation of the case, there are numerous other specialty views and techniques that can be performed to gain additional information. As stated previously, a detailed lameness examination is also required to guide the practitioner in deciding what radiographic views should be taken. Radiography is also very useful in more thorough evaluation of the sound horse's foot for consultation with the farrier with respect to trimming and shoeing protocols. Although DR has improved the ability to visualize and evaluate some of the soft tissue structures within the foot, there remain great limitations to imaging most soft tissue structures within the foot.

REFERENCES

1. McKnight AL. Digital radiography in equine practice. Clin Tech Equine Pract 2004;3:352–60.
2. S. Dyson Lameness and diagnostic imaging in the sports horse: recent advances related to the digit. In: Proceedings. Florida: American Association of Equine Practitioners; 2007;53. p. 262–75.
3. Redden RF. Radiographic imaging of the equine foot. Vet Clin North Am Equine Pract 2003;19:379–92, vi.
4. Caudron I, Miesen M, Grulke S, et al. Radiological assessment of the effects of a full rolling motion shoe during asymmetrical bearing. Equine Vet J Suppl 1997;23:20–2.
5. Butler JA, Colles CM, Dyson SJ, et al. General principles. In: Clinical radiology of the horse. 3rd edition. Ames (IA): Wiley-Blackwell; 2008. p. 1–35.
6. Butler JA, Colles CM, Dyson SJ, et al. Computed and digital radiography. In: Clinical radiology of the horse. 3rd edition. Ames (IA): Wiley-Blackwell; 2008. p. 37–51.
7. Drost WT, Reese DJ, Hornof WJ. Digital radiography artifacts. Vet Radiol Ultrasound 2008;49:S48–56.
8. Jimenez DA, Armbrust LJ, O'Brien RT, et al. Artifacts in digital radiography. Vet Radiol Ultrasound 2008;49:321–32.
9. Little DR, Schramme M. Diagnostic imaging: radiography and radiology of the foot. In: Floyd AE, Mansmann RA, editors. Equine podiatry. St Louis (MO): Saunders-Elsevier; 2007. p. 141–59.
10. Kummer M, Geyer H, Imboden I, et al. The effect of hoof trimming on radiographic measurements of the front feet of normal Warmblood horses. Vet J 2006;172:58–66.
11. Cripps PJ, Eustace RA. Radiological measurements from the feet of normal horses with relevance to laminitis. Equine Vet J 1999;31:427–32.

12. Kummer M, Gygax D, Lischer C, et al. Comparison of the trimming procedure of six different farriers by quantitative evaluation of hoof radiographs. Vet J 2009; 179:401–6.

13. Van Heel MC, Moleman M, Barneveld A, et al. Changes in location of centre of pressure and hoof-unrollment pattern in relation to an 8-week shoeing interval in the horse. Equine Vet J 2005;37:536–40.

14. A. Smith S. Dyson R. Murray Is there an association between distal phalanx angles and deep digital flexor tendon lesions? In: Proceedings. Denver(CO): American Association of Equine Practitioners; 2004;50. p. 328–31.

15. Page BT, Hagen TL. Breakover of the hoof and its effect on structures and forces within the foot. J Equine Vet Sc 2002;22:258–64.

16. Eliashar E, McGuigan MP, Wilson AM. Relationship of foot conformation and force applied to the navicular bone of sound horses at the trot. Equine Vet J 2004;36: 431–5.

17. Verschooten F, Roels J, Lampo P, et al. Radiographic measurement from the lateromedial projection of the equine foot with navicular disease. Res Vet Sci 1989; 46:15–21.

18. Dyson SJ, Tranquille CA, Collins SN, et al. An investigation of the relationships between angles and shapes of the hoof capsule and the distal phalanx. Equine Vet J 2011;43:295–301.

19. Linford RL, O'Brien TR, Trout DR. Qualitative and morphometric radiographic findings in the distal phalanx and digital soft tissues of sound thoroughbred racehorses. Am J Vet Res 1993;54:38–51.

20. Parks A. Form and function of the equine digit. Vet Clin North Am Equine Pract 2003;19:285–307, v.

21. O'Grady SE. Radiographs for the farrier. Therapeutic Farriery and Equine Podiatry Consulting Service 2003. Available at: http://www.equipodiatry.com/index.html.

22. Parks A. The foot and shoeing. In: Ross MW, Dyson SJ, editors. Diagnosis and management of lameness in the horse. 2nd edition. St Louis (MO): Elsevier-Saunders; 2011. p. 282–302.

23. Dik KJ. Role of navicular bone shape in the pathogenesis of navicular disease: a radiological study. Equine Vet J 1995;27:390–3.

24. Dyson S. Radiological interpretation of the navicular bone. Equine Vet Educ 2008; 20:268–80.

25. Merritt K. How to take foot radiographs. In: Proceedings. San Diego(CA): American Association of Equine Practitioners; 2008;54. p. 233–9.

The Basics of Farriery as a Prelude to Therapeutic Farriery

Hans H. Castelijns, DVM, CF

KEYWORDS

- Farriery • Hoof trimming • Therapeutic shoeing • Horseshoe types
- Horseshoe nails

KEY POINTS

- Domesticated horses need hoof care, because it is rare for the wear and growth of the hooves to be in perfect equilibrium.
- During the shoeing interval, the hoof grows downwards and forward in the direction of the horn tubules, losing some degree of angle.
- Few horses have perfect limb conformation. The shape of a hoof of a limb with conformation defects adapts in a predictable way to these defects.
- If, for therapeutic or performance reasons, the hoof-shoe combination is modified, there is not a lot of leeway in the trim of a particular foot, whereas the applied shoe type, placement, and adjustments provide endless possibilities.

INTRODUCTION

The terms, *farriery* and *farrier*, derive from the French, *ferrer* (to shoe), and include the root, *fer* (iron). The French term for farrier, however, is *maréchal ferrant*, wherein *maréchal* means officer (general), and *ferrant* means one who shoes. Equine veterinary text books from the Middle Ages often have marechaucie, marescallie, or mariescalla in their titles, both denoting the importance of farriery and the fact that the equine veterinarian and farrier often were one and the same and even of noble birth.[1] The technique of nailing an iron (steel) shoe onto a hoof is currently the most economic form of hoof protection as far as material costs go, because the metal is cheap. In the Gallo-Roman period and in the Middle Ages, however, mining ore and forging iron into horseshoes were a luxury, only justifiable with the need to efficiently protect the feet of valuable horses, especially the heavy warhorse.[2] The points of this historical etymological recall are that (1) farriery had enormous importance at the time when horses were immensely valuable (a warhorse could cost as much as a farm) and (2) shoeing was and is sometimes the only way to allow a horse to function in the service of humans.

The author has nothing to disclose.
Loc. Valecchie 11/A, Cortona 52040, AR, Italy
E-mail address: hansdomi@tin.it

Vet Clin Equine 28 (2012) 313–331
http://dx.doi.org/10.1016/j.cveq.2012.06.003
0749-0739/12/$ – see front matter © 2012 Published by Elsevier Inc.

THE TRIM

Domesticated horses need hoof care, because it is rare for the wear and growth of the hooves to be in perfect equilibrium. When the quality of the hooves (size in relationship to body mass, sole depth, wall thickness, quality of intertubular horn, and so forth) is good, the footing favorable, and the workload not excessive, horses can, and should, generally be left barefoot. An exception is poor conformation; for example, an important angular limb deviation may cause excessive, asymmetric wear and growth across an otherwise strong hoof and certain pathologies. An example of this is a horse affected with bone spavin that may wear the outside of its hind hooves excessively.

The Barefoot Trim

Trimming the feet of a horse that does not need shoes is not different from trimming for shoeing, except that the horny sole should be left intact and the hooves, specifically the walls, should be left slightly longer (3–5 mm) and the outside edges rounded off at a radius of at least half the wall thickness (**Fig. 1**). Rounding the outside edge of the toe slightly more may be indicated for those horses that live on dry, hard (that is, impenetrable) ground. If a horse lives on wet, deep ground, it might be useful to leave slightly more toe wall to keep it from sinking in too much.

Trimming the Foot for Shoes

During the shoeing interval, the hoof grows downwards and forward in the direction of the horn tubules, losing some degree of angle relative to the ground, as seen from the side, **Fig. 2**A because the heels, with their lateromedial movement on the rigid shoe surface, continue to wear (**Fig. 2**B).[3] It is, therefore, important to keep shoeing intervals short (5–6 weeks, depending on growth rate) and regular.[4] The basic trim should commence by identifying the true apex of the frog and removing the adjacent defoliating sole until the compact nonexfoliating sole horn is reached because this identifies the appropriate sole depth. This is followed by removing the exfoliated sole from the remainder of the ground surface of the foot, including the sole between the bars and the heels (seat of corn), all the way to the white line (**Fig. 3**). The rest of the frog is then trimmed only enough to guard the triangular shape with its small central cleft, which forms the ideal breaking, shock-absorbing, and expansion organ, as seen in transverse section (**Fig. 4**). A light trim of the lateral and medial body of the frog is also

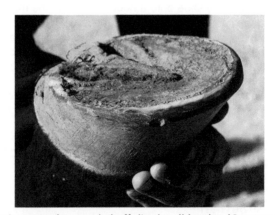

Fig. 1. Barefoot trim; note the rounded off distal wall border. (*Courtesy of* Hans H. Castelijns, DVM, CF, Cortona, Italy.)

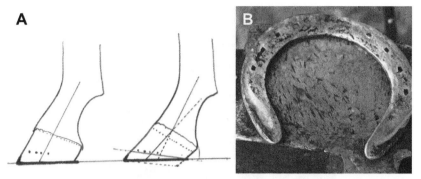

Fig. 2. (*A*) Schematic presentation of the barely shod hoof and 8 weeks later; although both the toe and the heels grow (dotted line, parallel to the coronary band) only the heels continue to wear, the result is that the digital axis is broken back. (*B*) Wear marks on the upper heel surface of the shoe: if the heels on the upper surface of the steel shoe are worn, how much heel of the foot has been worn down? (*Courtesy of* Hans H. Castelijns, DVM, CF, Cortona, Italy.)

important to make (self) cleaning of the corresponding sulci possible, especially of the shod hoof.

After the sole trim, the excess hoof wall length is easy to judge and easy to trim. The sole, however, follows the slight cup of the distal phalanx, not only in the lateromedial sense but also in the dorsopalmar (plantar) sense, so if the trimmed ground surface of the hoof is to be flat, to accommodate the application of a flat shoe, the wall might slightly protrude from the trimmed sole plane at the level of the quarters (**Fig. 5**). The bars should be even with the wall at the heels, at least where they contact the shoe, so as to be weight bearing, because otherwise the weight, on the upper surface of the heels of the shoe, is only borne by the heel wall. Ideally the wall should be trimmed back to the widest part of the frog, compatible with the sole depth at the

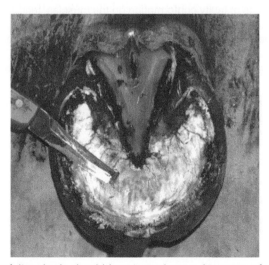

Fig. 3. Only the exfoliated sole should be trimmed away. (*Courtesy of* Hans H. Castelijns, DVM, CF, Cortona, Italy.)

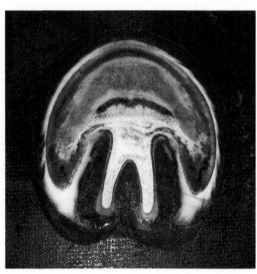

Fig. 4. Section of the foot parallel to the coronary band; note how the frog and digital cushion form an expansion organ in the caudal part. (*Courtesy of* Hans H. Castelijns, DVM, CF, Cortona, Italy.)

seat of corn, because this increases the foot's surface and, therefore, dispersion of pressure in the delicate palmar/plantar area (**Fig. 6**).[5]

HOOF CAPSULE DISTORTION VERSUS ADAPTATION IN FORM
Hoof Capsule Adaptation to Limb Conformation

Few horses have perfect limb conformation. The shape of a hoof of a limb with conformation defects adapts in a predictable way to these defects (as does the shape of the distal phalanx[6]). This adaptation in hoof shape serves the horse well, because it limits the deleterious effects of faulty conformation on the muscles, tendons, ligaments, and joints. In the sagittal plane, conformation defects can best be described as hyperextensions (more than normal extension or dorsiflexion) or hypoextensions (less than normal extension or flexion) of the joints, as seen from the side. The shape of the hoof, as seen from the side, for example, depends mainly on the tension of the

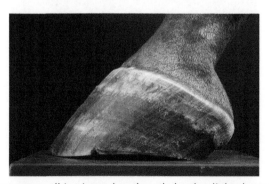

Fig. 5. When the quarter wall is trimmed to the sole level, a light dorsopalmar cup forms, which does not easily accommodate a flat shoe. (*Courtesy of* M. Savoldi.)

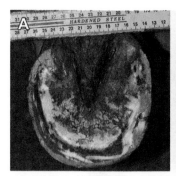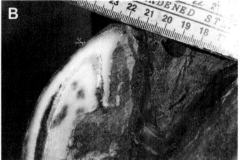

Fig. 6. (*A, B*) The heels, when trimmed to the largest part of the frog, increase the caudal surface area of the hoof. (*Courtesy of* Hans H. Castelijns, DVM, CF, Cortona, Italy.)

deep digital flexor tendon (and the integrity of the dorsal laminar apparatus), which determines the palmar, plantar angle of the distal phalanx. Too much tension and there is clubfoot (flexion of the distal interphalangeal [DIP]) joint with an upright dorsal wall angle, a narrow short toe, and long strong heels. In the adult horse with this condition, the limited capacity for extension in its DIP joint (dorsiflexion) is best served by this hoof shape, which facilitates quick breakover.

In the frontal plane, abnormal conformation is described as valgus (the limb's segment distal to the affected joint deviating laterally) or varus (the distal segment deviating medially). Again, as an example, the shape of the ground surface of a hoof of a limb with a metacarpophalangeal/metatarsophalangeal varus is narrower laterally and wider medially, which again serves the horse well because it diminishes excessive lateral torque on the proximal interphalangeal (PIP) joint and DIP joint, which in this conformation are not parallel to the ground.

In the horizontal plane, conformation abnormalities are characterized by axial rotations of the limb or its segments, either outwards or inwards. Thus, choosing again a frequently encountered defect, this time in the horizontal plane, a limb with a medial (inward) rotation of the digit relative to the metacarpus/metatarsus bone develops a hoof with a diagonal asymmetry, with a narrow lateral toe and medial heel and a wide medial toe and lateral heel (**Fig. 7**). This wry, perhaps unpleasing, hoof shape again offers some biomechanical advantages, aligning the 2 heels on landing and diminishing the lever arm on breakover, because with this conformation the interphalangeal joints are not hinged at 90° to the direction of movement of the horse or its body midline (**Fig. 8**).[7] A single limb may, and often does, present several conformational defects, each adding its influence on the shape and outline of the hoof. Although this may render the interpretation of the hoof shape harder, it follows the same logic, that is, the overburdened parts of the hoof are less developed whereas the less burdened parts overdevelop. The frequent combination, for example, of an inwardly rotated digit combined with a varus fetlock in the same limb results in a hoof with an asymmetric toe (because both conditions shrink the outside toe) but more symmetric heels (as in the heel area, the 2 different conformation defects tend to even out their influence on the hoof).

The conclusion that a crooked limb is best served by an asymmetric hoof shape is supported not only by theoretic biomechanical considerations but also by a thorough doctoral research project, which resulted in more than 10 peer-reviewed articles.[8] Especially interesting is the finding that in a dorsopalmar radiograph of the digit, joint spacing should be even, although the distal phalanx may not be parallel to the ground, that is, with an asymmetric hoof shape. Also noteworthy is the discovery that a correct

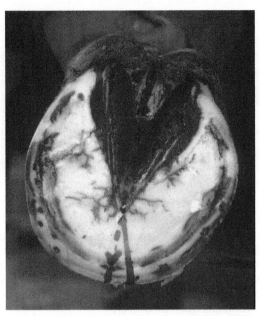

Fig. 7. Right fore with an inwardly rotated digit; the midline of the frog and the hoof capsule (*dotted line*) are rotated relative to the direction of movement (*straight line*). Note the atrophy (smaller size) of the medial heel and lateral toe, which is where landing, respectively breakover, take place compared with the lateral heel and medial toe. (*Courtesy of* Hans H. Castelijns, DVM, CF, Cortona, Italy.)

protocol is needed to take meaningful dorsopalmar radiographs to evaluate lateromedial joint spacing and phalangeal alignment and rotation. It is, furthermore, an old and respectable principle of farriery to shape the shoe to the (asymmetric) foot and not to trim the foot to fit the (symmetric) shoe.

Hoof Capsule Distortion and Correction

Abnormal limb conformation leads to hoof shape adaptation, but asymmetric ground reaction force on the hoof, due to uneven landing, weight bearing, and propulsion,

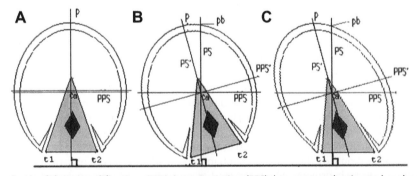

Fig. 8. Hoof shape modification, DIP joint orientation (PPS), lever arm reduction to breakover point (pb), and heel alignment (t_1, t_2), in the case of axial rotation of the digit (p). (*A*) Schematic hoof with no axial rotation. (*B*) Axial rotation without hoofshape adaptation. (*C*) Axial rotation with hoofshape modification. (*Courtesy of* Hans H. Castelijns, DVM, CF, Cortona, Italy.)

can also easily lead to hoof capsule distortion. Distinguishing between the 2 is at the heart of preventive shoeing because distortion should be corrected whereas adaptation of hoof shape should not. True hoof capsule distortion is characterized by bent horn tubules. Under excessive, repetitive strain, the distal part of the horn tubules in the dorsal part of the hoof bends outward, causing a flare. In the palmar/plantar part of the hoof, however, the distal part of the tubules bends inward or even forward at the heels (under run heels). The explanation of the apparently different responses, depending on location, is that on landing, with the limb protracted, the hoof wall in the heel area is compressed toward the inside of the foot, whereas during breakover the dorsal wall is pulled away from the center. Thus, in the example of the inward axial rotation of the digit, the 2 atrophied areas of the hoof (lateral toe and medial heel) distort differently. The outside toe wall flattens and flares out; the medial heel wall becomes steeper, and its distal part might even bend inwards (roll under). Another, related form of distortion may occur in the palmar/plantar area of the hoof and is characterized by upward displacement of the coronary band, because the affected quarter heel may shunt upward under excessive load, especially when the wall here is vertical or rolled under.[9]

An upwardly sheared heel may not leave enough free margin of the ungual cartilage above the coronary band for its normal abaxial movement under load, which in the author's experience predisposes the horse to developing a quarter crack. Hoof distortion correction, appropriate and necessary, is done by removing flares of the dorsal hoof wall with the rasp until there is a straight line from the coronary band to the distal border of the hoof. In the heel area, a distortion is addressed by a double trim method. First the foot is trimmed to keep the joint spacing even in the lateromedial aspect. As seen from the side, the aim is to keep a straight pastern dorsal hoof wall alignment. A second trim is then performed on the side of the under-rolled, upwardly shunted heel, starting at the toe and running in a straight line all the way to heel, ideally going from 0 mm at the toe to as many millimeters as are needed to take away at the heel to give it the same length as the contralateral heel of the same foot. On nailing on the shoe, the upwardly shunted heel then settles down onto the shoe, eliminating the space created by the second trim. The lowered coronary band then frees up space for the ipsilateral ungual cartilage to expand on weight bearing. The free margin, above the proximal border of the hoof wall, of the ungular cartilage should be a minimum of 15 mm on an average-sized foot (**Fig. 9**).[10]

The second trim usually removes most of the under-rolled distal heel wall, which on settling down also moves slightly outwards (abaxially), lessening the verticality of this area of the wall (**Fig. 10**).

INSTRUMENTAL AIDS FOR TRIMMING

Because outward marks of the foot (uniform sole depth, widest part of the frog, apex of the frog, hoof pastern alignment, horn tubule direction, and so forth) are not always easy to interpret in horses with limb conformation abnormalities, and because few horses have perfect limbs, the use of some instruments may aid the trimming process.

Radiographic imagining is discussed in the article by Eggleston elsewhere in this issue; however, to get a dorsopalmar horizontal radiograph that is usable for trimming measurements, a special protocol should be used.[8]

The foot should be placed on a rotating radiograph block, the opposite foot lifted up, and the x-ray beam aligned with the sagittal plane of the foot. To obtain this, a linear metal marker is placed onto, and aligned with, the central horn tubule. Only those horizontal DP foot radiographs on which the marker is aligned with the central cleft of the frog can be used for accurate joint space analysis. Even joint spacing should be the

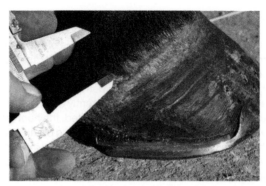

Fig. 9. The ungular cartilage should have a palpable free margin, above the coronary band, of at least 15 mm; otherwise, a quarter crack may occur. (*Courtesy of* Hans H. Castelijns, DVM, CF, Cortona, Italy.)

aim of the trim in the lateromedial sense. The central horn tubule can be found by aligning the central frog cleft with a point at the toe; the horn tubule at the dorsal wall that hits this point is the central one. In many feet, especially front feet, this point coincides with a black grayish interruption of the white line, which denotes the presence of the crena marginalis (notch of the dorsodistal border) of the distal phalanx.

Fortunately, the Caudron's study concluded that in the overwhelming majority of cases, the same trimming results could be obtained with the use of a Finnegan hoof gauge (Equine Hoof Management, Rocklin, California), whereby the bottom of the foot is trimmed at 90° to the direction of the central horn tubule (**Fig. 11**). When using this instrument, it is essential to keep the bottom slit of the gauge aligned with the central cleft and apex of the frog. If the dorsal slit corresponds and is aligned with the central horn tubule, the lateromedial trim allows for even joint spacing of the interphalangeal joints.

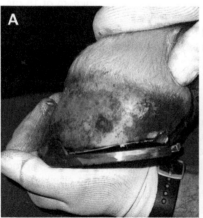
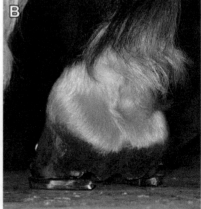

Fig. 10. Right hind. (*A*) To lower the sheared medial heel, a "wedge" is cut away after the basic trim; the important detail is to start the second trim at the toe. (*B*) When the shoe is then nailed on and the foot set down, the gap disappears, because the medial wall settles down. Notice the good alignment of the bulbs. (*Courtesy of* Hans H. Castelijns, DVM, CF, Cortona, Italy.)

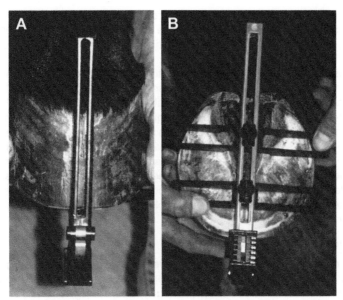

Fig. 11. (A, B) Use of the Finnegan hoof gauge: the bottom of the hoof should ideally be at 90° to the central horn tubule. (*Courtesy of* Hans H. Castelijns, DVM, CF, Cortona, Italy.)

SHOEING

It is the author's conviction that, except for horses with particular severe foot conditions, like laminitis, "the foot tells us how it should be trimmed" (discussed previously in the section on trimming). If, for therapeutic or performance reasons, the hoof-shoe combination is modified, there is a not a lot of leeway in the trim of a particular foot, whereas the applied shoe type, placement, and adjustments provide endless possibilities. A practical example of this principle is therapeutic shoeing for podotrocleosis (navicular disease or palmar foot pain). In a typical patient, dorsiflexion (extension) of the DIP joint is limited due to the pathology. Theoretically it makes sense to limit the dorsiflexion of the DIP joint by leaving the heels longer.[11] In practice, however, there is upward displacement of the walls at the heels[10]; a shorter, often underrun, solar surface of the palmar part of the hoof; more heel wear on the branches of the shoe; and a different stance of the horse as seen from the side, with the horse placing its front limbs further back, under itself. In the author's experience, however, the same case can be treated without these collateral effects by trimming the heels to the widest part of the frog (as discussed previously) and then shoeing at short, regular intervals with a shoe that facilitates dorsal breakover (blunt toe shoe, reverse shoe, rockered toe shoe, and so forth).

General Principles

No matter what the final performance or therapeutic aim, some general principles apply to all or most shoe applications:

- Only shoe when necessary, that is, when wear and tear are more than the hoof can bear, when shoes are part of necessary treatment, or when horses need shoes for traction.
- The trim is the most important part of a shoeing job; flares and sheared heels should be corrected. The hoof should be short and proportioned, because it only grows longer and forward before the next shoeing.

- The shoe should be shaped to the foot and the nail holes should correspond to the white line: nail too coarsely and there may be compression or infection of the solar, white line or laminar corium; nail too fine and the wall will break apart over time.
- Choose the appropriate materials: the choice of shoe depends on the horse, hoof shape and quality (like hoof wall thickness), type of work, and footing. There is no single shoe type that is appropriate for all horses and all disciplines. The type of nail depends on the type of shoe, hoof quality, and type of work but in any case the type, number, and placement of nails should assure that it is the weakest link; in the case of shoe loss, no part of the wall should come away with the shoe.
- The best shoeing job looks and functions poorly if the shoes are left on too long. Respect shoeing intervals first and foremost and allow for appropriate shoe width and length at the heels, because the foot grows forward and widens between shoeing appointments. After a reasonable shoeing interval, the shoe should still cover the wall at the heels.

Performance, Prevention, and Therapy

A detailed discussion on the relationship between performance and shoeing is outside the scope of this article. Shoeing influence on performance is closely related to the discipline the horse is used in. Examples are gaited horses (eg, Icelandic and Tennessee Walking), trotters, and pacers. If a racing trotter has a tendency to pace during acceleration, the 3 shoeing modifications that might prevent this are heavier shoes, longer toes, and more grip. None of these is necessarily healthy. Sometimes an equine practitioner is called on to rein in excessive enthusiasm of trainer and farrier for extreme solutions that are perceived as performance enhancing. The definitive argument is that a lame horse does not perform at all.

Prevention is related to both discipline and therapy because some sports are associated with specific injuries and prevention of (re)injury is better than (re)treating a lameness.

THERAPEUTIC SHOEING WAYS AND MEANS

The basic therapeutic shoeing means at the disposal of the equine podiatrist are

1. Breakover modifications (eg, rockered toe)
2. Ground surface modifications of the shoe (eg, egg bar shoe)
3. Modifications of hoof support and weight bearing (eg, the use of hoof packing or of a heart bar)
4. Shock-absorbing shoeing (pads or plastic shoes).
5. Weight reduction (eg, aluminum shoes)
6. Hoof wall defect stabilization (eg, quarter crack repair with patches or glue on shoes)

Most of these means can be, and often are, combined in the treatment of a specific pathology.

Breakover Modifications

Dorsal breakover is defined as the moment the heels lift off the ground in the last part of the stance phase. In a horse moving straight, with normal conformation and on a flat hard surface, the fulcrum (breakover point) is not the center of the toe but slightly lateral of this point,[12] at least on the front feet. In a limb that presents conformation abnormalities, such as axial rotations or angular deviations, the point of breakover varies, even when moving on a straight line on flat hard ground. Thus, a toed-out conformation causes the point of breakover to change toward the center or even the medial part of the toe. Even more markedly, a toed-in horse clearly breaks over the outside toe. On deep ground, the same force pulling the distal phalanx out of its most extended position into flexion, that is, the deep digital flexor tendon, finds less resistance because the toe of the shoe can "roll" into the ground.

When a horse is turning or when it travels on uneven ground, the fulcrum is again modified; on a right hand turn, the left fore breaks over at the medial toe, the right fore over the lateral one. On an individual horse, the average point of breakover is worn on the ground surface of the shoe, at a specific area of the toe. It is good, preventive farriery practice to roll or rocker the toe at this same point on the new shoe.

The anatomic structures that are solicited most in the last part of the stance phase, just before breakover, are the deep digital flexor tendon, its accessory ligament (inferior check ligament), the collateral ligaments of the distal sesamoid, the navicular bursa, the impar ligament, the dorsal laminae, the dorsal aspects of the carpal joints, and the dorsal margins of the DIP joint. When the last phase of the stance phase occurs on a sharp turn, as when a show jumper changes direction toward the next obstacle, the collateral ligaments of the navicular bone, DIP joint, PIP joint, metacarpophalangeal joint, and even the suspensory branch opposite to the side of the turn are stressed, as is the subcondral bone of the joints on the side of the direction change.

Facilitating dorsal breakover can be done by setting back the shoe relative to the toe of the trimmed hoof, blunting the toe of the shoe, rolling the ground surface of the shoe in the toe area, rockering it, or a combination of all four (**Fig. 12**). Facilitating sideways breakover can be done by choosing shoes with a narrowed ground surface all around their perimeter, like some concave shoes, half-round section shoes, or full rolling motion shoes (**Fig. 13**).[13] A simple and effective way to facilitate dorsal, lateral, and medial breakover is the French rockered shoe. In the French (and Swiss) tradition, sport horses are routinely shod with a rocker toe shoe, which starts at the second or third nail hole and goes around the toe, all the way to the opposite toe or even quarter. In this type of rockered shoe, the inside ground edge of the shoe should still be on the anvil (or ground of the shod foot). The dorsal part of the shoe does, therefore, look like a dish or bowl. Apart from offering multidirectional ease of breakover, this shoeing method also gives sole relief (because the inside foot edge of the shoe is forged down with a hammer) and improves nail pitch. Flexible shoes, like plastic shoes or flaps (**Fig. 14**), also maintain vertical flexibility in the hoof, absorbing a few degrees of the inclination in the hoof capsule, instead of in the joints, on a sharp direction change of the horse.

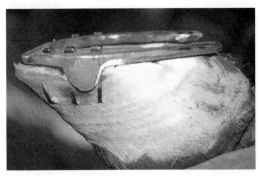

Fig. 12. A combination of rockered, rolled, and setback toe facilitates dorsal breakover; the nail heads have to be filed down. (*Courtesy of* Hans H. Castelijns, DVM, CF, Cortona, Italy.)

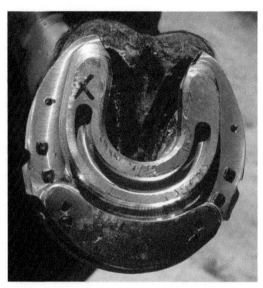

Fig. 13. Full rolling motion shoes facilitate lateral and medial breakover the most. (*Courtesy of* Hans H. Castelijns, DVM, CF, Cortona, Italy.)

The use of a digital extension device (DED) permits the exact measurement of the tolerance to dorsal extension and lateral and medial elevation (and even flexion) on the standing horse of each (front) limb on both a sound horse and a lame horse (**Fig. 15**). The value of this test is not as much diagnostic as it is indicative of the specific type of therapeutic shoeing that is most effective, because, for example, a reduced tolerance to dorsal extension may depend on many different lesions. It predicts which therapeutic shoe will help (**Table 1**).

A study of 250 sound horses, freshly shod or trimmed, gave the following values: dorsal extension (mean 43.18° ± 0.93°; 95% CI); lateral elevation (mean 18.83° ± 0.26°); and medial elevation (mean 19.79° ± 0.32°). The standard deviations were 7.46°, 2.12°, and 2.53°, respectively.[14]

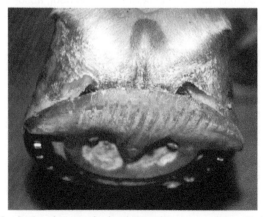

Fig. 14. Flaps are shock absorbing in the heel area. (*Courtesy of* Hans H. Castelijns, DVM, CF, Cortona, Italy.)

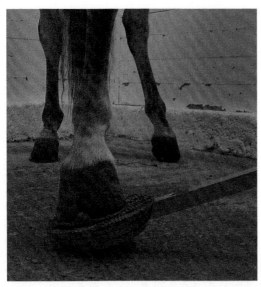

Fig. 15. Lateral elevation with the DED; maximum elevation is reached when the opposite side of the hoof lifts of the board. (*Courtesy of* Hans H. Castelijns, DVM, CF, Cortona, Italy.)

To illustrate the correlation between the hypothetical result of a digital extension test and the therapeutic shoeing needs of a hypothetical patient, the following example may be useful: if the right fore lame limb shows 28° of tolerance to dorsal extension, 15° of lateral elevation, and 19° of medial elevation (before the opposite side of the hoof lifts off the board), the hoof of the right fore needs a therapeutic shoe that facilitates dorsal and lateral breakover, for example, a shoe with a setback, blunted, and rolled toe and with the lateral ground surface ground away.

Ground Surface Modifications

As opposed to breakover modifications, which have an effect on both compact and penetrable ground (although they may be more necessary on compact ground), ground surface modifications, such as wide-webbed heels, toes, or branches of the shoe, have most of their effect on penetrable ground. A wide-webbed toe and narrow-heeled shoe (**Fig. 16**) prevents the toe from sinking into the ground at the midstance phase in deep footing, but on hard ground this shoe acts no differently from a normal shoe (placed in the same position). To give an example in the opposite sense, an egg bar shoe prevents heel sinking, relative to a normal shoe, only on penetrable ground.

On penetrable footing, the modifications of the ground surface of the shoe (and its placement relative to the trimmed foot) change the center of ground reaction force in all 3 moments of the stance phase, sometimes with unintended consequences.

At speed, horses land heel first, soliciting the back part of the foot and its shock-absorbing function and also straining the digital extensor tendon and its distal insertions (**Fig. 17**). In the midstance phase, with the fetlock at maximum extension, the suspensory ligament and the superficial digital flexor tendon are at peak tension. At the end of the stance phase, just before breakover, the distal deep digital flexor tendon (and other structures discussed previously) is at peak stress.[15] Thus, an egg bar shoe with a setback blunted toe, favors the sinking in of the toe on penetrable footing,

Table 1
Summary of therapeutic shoeing techniques in relationship to diagnosis, DED test results, and surface the horse works on

Condition: DIP, PIP Arthrosis, and/or Podotrocleosis	Intolerance to (DED Test)	Works on Surface	Shoeing, Trimming Techniques
Single collateral ligament lesion, single lobe of distal DDFT single collateral ligament of DS	Lateral or medial elevation	Deep	Narrow-webbed shoe, beveled ground surface on the side of intolerance, wider ground surface on the opposite side, short hooves, short shoeing intervals
		Compact	1. Flexible shoes (eg, flaps, easy walker) 2. Strongly beveled ground surface (outside rim) on the side of intolerance 3. Rockered ipsilateral toe shoe (French rockered toe), full rolling motion shoes, slightly displaced toward the opposite side of the intolerance 4. Note: short intervals; do not leave heels too long/high, especially in the case of dorsal entheseophytes
DIP arthrosis	Lateral and medial	Deep	1. Short, barefoot trim, well-rounded borders, not too much heel 2. Flexible shoes, short shoeing intervals 3. Half-round section shoes, tightly fit (eg, classic roller or eventer)
		Compact	1. French rockered toe (rocker goes from quarter over the toe to opposite quarter; heels stay flat) 2. Half-round section shoes 3. Full rolling motion shoes (eg, rock 'n roll, PG shoes); note: consider shock absorption (aluminum, pads), keep shoeing intervals short, do not set the shoes too wide
Navicular bursitis, distal DDF, tendonitis, impar ligament desmitis	Dorsal extension	Deep	1. Rolled-rockered-setback toe shoes 2. The same plus egg bar 3. Reverse shoeing
		Compact	1. Rolled-rockered toe 2. Blunt—setback toe (eg, NBS or sagittal, aluminum, square toed (wear is faster in the toe between shoeing intervals) 3. Shock-absorbing pads, mild frog support pads (test for sensibility of the frog area) 4. Full rolling motion shoes with the ground area at the toe strongly beveled; the higher total thickness of the shoe permits an extreme rolled toe
DIP arthrosis and podotrocleosis	Dorsal extension and lateral and medial elevation	Deep	1. Setback shoe (blunt toe) with beveled ground edges and egg bar 2. Palmar frog and sole support (less heel penetration) 3. Full rolling motion shoe with heel bar
		Compact	1. Full rolling motion shoe, with small central base, well set back 2. Shock-absorbing pad if sensitive to hammer blows to the shoe, short shoeing intervals

Abbreviations: DDF, deep digital fl...; or DDFT, deep digital flexor tendon; DS, ...; NBS, ...

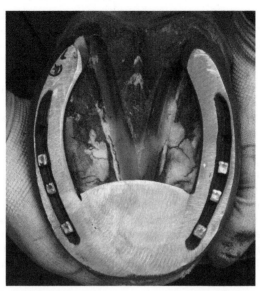

Fig. 16. A wide-webbed toe and narrow-heeled shoe prevents the toe from sinking into the ground, which would exaggerate fetlock extension in the midstance phase. (*Courtesy of* Loic Entwistle, Windesheim, Germany.)

facilitating breakover, relieving the deep digital flexor tendon. Alternatively, in the mid-stance phase, it might excessively strain the suspensory ligament and superficial digital flexor tendon more. On landing, the palmar part of the egg bar causes more of a pull on the distal insertion of the digital extension tendon. Briefly, "there is no free lunch"; when relieving one anatomic structure, during a particular phase of the stance, other structures are charged more in the other stance phases.

Modifications of Hoof Support and Weight Bearing

One of the drawbacks of a classical, nailed-on, open shoe is that it distances the sole, frog, and part of the bars from the ground, thereby reducing the weight-bearing parts of the hoof to the walls and ultimately to the laminar suspensory apparatus.

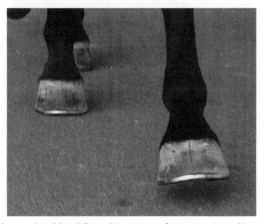

Fig. 17. At speed, horses land heel first. (*Courtesy of* Hans H. Castelijns, DVM, CF, Cortona, Italy.)

Many hoof conditions, such as weak and underrun heels, hoof wall defects, laminitis, and so forth, can benefit from recruiting the bars, frog, or parts of these, into weight bearing. Special shoes that have this function are the heart bar shoe and the onion heel shoe, which recruit the frog and the bars, respectively, into weight bearing (**Figs. 18** and **19**).

Specialty pads, with or without fast-setting hoof packing materials, can also have this function, besides having shock-absorbing properties. Sole packing materials are distinguished by different hardness, chemical composition, weight, wear resistance, setting times, adhesiveness to the sole, ability to perspire, and application method.[16]

Pads and sole packing can also be used to protect thin soles against bruises, especially the softer, lightweight ones. When applying a sole packing, it is useful to do a check on the tolerance to pressure of the frog, remembering that the overlaying structures include the digital cushion, deep digital flexor tendon, navicular bursa, and distal sesamoid, all of which can be inflamed and painful. Care must also be taken when applying sole packing over a frog with thrush. This check can be done with hoof testers or by placing the frog on a wooden handle and lifting up the opposite foot. A positive (pain) reaction should counsel the use of soft packing material.

Shock-Absorbing Shoeing

Shock and high-frequency vibrations are implicated in pain, ischemia, and osteoarthritic degeneration, similar to white finger syndrome in humans. A useful clinical sign is when the horse is uncomfortable with the hammer blows while driving the nails when setting a shoe. Horses that often benefit from shock-absorbing shoeing are those, such as harness or carriage horses, that are called on to work on hard surfaces.

Shock absorption can be achieved by interposing pads and sole packing between the shoe and the hoof or with specialty shoes that absorb shock on the ground surface. In the first case, it is important to drill holes in the pad, in correspondence

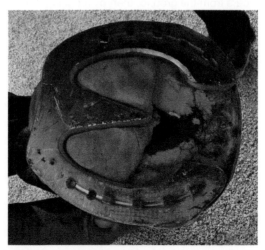

Fig. 18. Open toe, heart bar shoe with dental impression material in the palmar part of the hoof. (*Courtesy of* Hans H. Castelijns, DVM, CF, Cortona, Italy.)

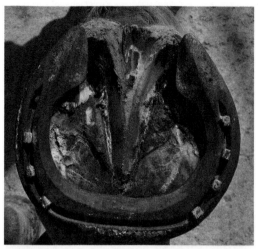

Fig. 19. Onion shoe—the enlarged foot surface of the shoe's heels recruits the bars of the hoof in to weight bearing. (*Courtesy of* Hans H. Castelijns, DVM, CF, Cortona, Italy.)

to the nail holes of the shoe, before nailing the shoe/pad combination to the foot, to preserve the micromovement of the pad independently from the nails.

The farriery industry is constantly coming out with specialty shoes with shock-absorbing claims, but objective, comparable data (at least to the barefoot and normally steel-shod foot) are often lacking. For many fast disciplines (racing, eventing, and so forth), many of these products are too bulky and/or too heavy. For working day horses, excessive wear and/or cost is also often a problem. A solution is offered by products that have a rigid half-shoe or metal insert at the toe, for stable nailing, and shock-absorbing flexibility in the heel area, such as flaps, Epona shoes (www. EponaShoe.com), and so forth, because they preserve vertical mobility at the heels.

Weight Reduction

Lightweight shoes, mainly aluminum alloy, are used for performance (eg, flat racing) but also have other preventive and therapeutic properties. Aluminum alloys absorb high-frequency vibrations better than steel on hard compact ground,[17] offer better grip on this type of surface, and cause less fatigue. They also make it possible to have asymmetric, wide-webbed, or bar shoes, without excessive (asymmetric) weight increase and they diminish the limb's deviations from the normal flight arch (**Fig. 20**). Medial or lateral deviations, out of the sagittal plane, of the flight arch of the shod hoof, are common in horses, which respectively toe out or toe in and which in the first case often causes interference injuries to the contralateral limb.

Weight reduction also reduces hyperflexion (and extension) of the limb in the air between stance phases, which might benefit patients with articular (eg, fetlock and carpus) and tendon or suspensory ligament lesions.

Hoof Wall Defects Stabilization, Repair, and Glue on Shoes

Many severe hoof conditions can be successfully treated with glues and polymers, which are addressed in the article by O'Grady, Pleasant and McKinley elsewhere in this issue.

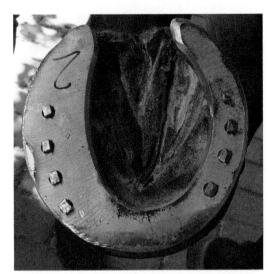

Fig. 20. Asymmetric shoes, in this case, with a wide lateral branch, have less asymmetric weight distribution if made out of aluminum alloys. (*Courtesy of* Hans H. Castelijns, DVM, CF, Cortona, Italy.)

SUMMARY

In most cases, therapeutic farriery depends on a correct trim (which is not necessarily the easiest part of farriery), because leaving extra length at one side of the hoof, at the heels, or at the toe leads to hoof capsule distortion. It is then that the type, placement, and modifications of the shoe make a (therapeutic) difference.

In lame horses, using a digital extension test may give valuable information regarding the most appropriate type of shoe for the specific lameness, because it lets the horse "speak for itself." This is especially important, because diagnostic capabilities have become more precise, often resulting in multiple diagnostic findings in the same limb, many of which might not be the cause of pain or diminished function.

When choosing the therapeutic features of a shoe/shoeing, it is useful to keep the type of horse, hooves, conformation, work, and surface on which the horse works in mind. The latter is important, because the therapeutic shoe/ground interaction is often at the heart of the success or failure of the intended podiatry treatment.

REFERENCES

1. Causati Vanni MA. Giordano Brusso nelle scuderie di Federico II imperatore ovvero, l'arte di curare il cavallo. Velettri (Rome): Editrice Vela; 2000. p. LVI–LIX.
2. D'Autherville P. Historique. In: Précis de Maréchalerie. Paris: Maloine S.A. Editeur; 1982. p. 15–20.
3. Craig M. The value of measuring the hoof. The Farriers Journal 2011;148:6–14.
4. Heel Van. M.C.V. "Changes in Location of center of pressure and hoof-unrollment pattern in relation to an 8 – week shoeing interval in the horse", chapter 5, "Distal Limb development and effects of shoeing techniques on limb dynamics of today's equine athlete". Doctoral thesis. Enschede (The Netherlands): Febodruk BV; 2005. p. 75–90.
5. Savoldi MT. Identifying the true foot of the horse, proceedings, 10th Geneva Congress of Equine Medicine and Surgery. December 11–13, 2007. p. 63–7.

6. Craig JJ, Craig MF, Burd M, et al. The palmar—metric: quantifying the quality of the equine distal phalange. The Farriers Journal 2011;149:8–22.

7. Castelijns HH. L'aplomb dans le plan diagonal, proceedings, 11ième Congrès Marèchaux et Vétérinaires, La Roche Sur Foron. January 28–30, 1999. p. 69–70.

8. Caudron J. Approche orthopédique des affections osteo-articulaires dégénératives de l'extrémité digitale du cheval, prévention et traitement. Doctoral thesis, Université de Liège, Faculté de Médecine Vétérinaire, 1997-1998.

9. O'Grady SE, Castelijns HH. Sheared heels and the correlation to spontaneous quarter cracks. Equine Vet Educ 2011;23(5):262–9.

10. Castelijns HH. Pathogenesis and treatment of spontaneous quarter cracks—quantifying vertical mobility of the hoof capsule at the heels, Pferdeheilkunde, 22 Jahrgang. 2006, Ausgabe 5, September – Oktober. p. 569–76.

11. Lawson SE, Château H, Pourcelot P, et al. Effect of toe and heel elevation on calculated tendon strains in the horse and the influence of the proximal interphalangeal joint. J Anat 2007;210:583–91.

12. Van Heel MC, Barneveld PR, Van Weeren PR, et al. Dynamic pressure measurement for the detailed study of hoof balance; the effect of trimming. Equine Vet J 2004;36(8):778–82.

13. Serteyn D, Vanschepdael P, Caudron I, et al. Evaluation Clinique de la ferrure orthopédique Equi+® Lors de pathologies de l'articulation interphalangienne distale. Pratique Vétérinaire Equine 1995;27(2):105–10 [in French].

14. Castelijns HH. How to use digital extension device in lameness examinations. 2008; vol. 54/AAEP Proceedings. p. 228–31.

15. Van Heel MC, Van Weeren PR, Back W. Shoeing sound Warmblood horses with a rolled-toe optimizes hoof unrollment and lowers peak loading during break over. Equine Vet J 2006;38(3):258–62.

16. Castelijns HH. Sole and frog support systems, proceeding 11th SIVE Congress. January 28–30, 2005. p. 52–5.

17. Benoit P, Barrey E, Regnault JC, et al. Comparison of the damping effect of different shoeing by the measurement of hoof acceleration. Acta Anat (Basel) 1993;146:109–13.

Therapeutic Farriery
One Veterinarian's Perspective

Andrew H. Parks, VetMB, MS, MRCVS

KEYWORDS

- Therapeutic farriery • Anatomy and function of horse shoes
- Application of shoeing principles

KEY POINTS

- There are only so many ways to modify the function of the foot with trimming and shoeing.
- The design of a horse shoe may often be modified to improve one aspect of foot function.
- Modifying a horse shoe to improve one aspect of foot function almost invariably impacts another aspect of foot function.
- The application of horse shoes may be based on a specific diagnosis or directed at a symptom.
- The application of shoeing principles is best approached using theoretical reasoning based on the research data that is available and experience.

INTRODUCTION

Therapeutic farriery is a common adjunct and sometimes mainstay in the treatment of many conditions of the foot. Ideally, the application of therapeutic farriery would follow a linear or algorithmic approach in which a definitive diagnosis determines which tissues are injured, and with this knowledge an optimal farriery solution can be applied. However, there are barriers to fulfilling both of these steps. With regards to the former, it is frequently not possible to arrive at a definitive diagnosis because either the equipment or expertise to make the diagnosis is not available, or because localization and imaging techniques have limitations that preclude a definitive diagnosis. In the case of the latter it is because there are significant gaps in our knowledge regarding how therapeutic farriery interventions affect the function of the structures of the foot. Fortunately, there has been considerable progress in both these areas so that they are becoming less and less of a barrier and the current understanding of the biomechanical basis underlying the function of the digit is described in detail in another article in this issue. In the meantime, clinicians must operate on the best available information, which with respect to farriery is largely based on

The author has nothing to disclose.
Department of Large Animal Medicine, College of Veterinary Medicine, University of Georgia, 501 DW Brooks Drive, Athens, GA 30602-7385, USA
E-mail address: parksa@uga.edu

extrapolation from scientific studies related to normal foot function and how shoes affect that, and personal experience.

Therapeutic shoeing is either directed at a specific diagnosis or at a symptom. As such there are overarching goals of treatment for each situation. When the diagnosis is specific, such as laminitis or navicular syndrome, the goals may be correspondingly well defined. However, treatment of symptoms may be more variable. For example, when lameness is the principal symptom, some horses may have corresponding hoof capsule distortions that may suggest a more clearly defined path of treatment, whereas others may not demonstrate any other symptoms and the treatment must be very generically based and a high degree of trial and error accepted. As such, goals form the conceptual basis of treatment. These goals may frequently be met in more than one way. Which implementation or objective is used is frequently based on veterinarian's or farrier's prior experience.

GOALS OF THERAPEUTIC SHOEING

The goals of therapeutic farriery should be considered as concepts that are applied to achieve the desired effect regardless of the manner in which they are achieved. The author recognizes at least 6 main variables that can be manipulated in the course of shoeing as variants from the most simple of patterns: (a) moderating concussion, (b) moving the center of pressure, (c) altering the distribution of force, (d) changing the ease of movement about the distal interphalangeal joint, (e) changing the traction between the shoe and ground, and (f) moderating the flight phase of the stride. Of these, some are heavily used in therapeutic shoeing, while others primarily used as performance enhancers and seldom used therapeutically (**Box 1**).

Moderating Concussion

The impact part of the stance phase is associated with high magnitude and frequency vibrations. The application of steel shoes increases the magnitude and frequency of shock waves experienced by the foot as it decelerates during the landing phase of the stride compared with an unshod foot.[1,2] Various shoe and shoe/pad combinations have been examined to determine if they can ameliorate the effect of impact. The evidence indicates that some specific shoes and shoe pad combinations can reduce the magnitude and frequency of impact vibrations, but other combinations do not.[1,3] In general, light synthetic shoes with a low stiffness and pads made of viscoelastic materials are the most effective. Unfortunately, except for those specifically tested in the literature, this information is not available for most shoes and pads.

Moving the Center of Pressure

The position of the center of pressure at any point in the stride determines the distribution of pressure between the medial and lateral, and the dorsal and palmar aspects of the foot. Whether it increases or decreases the stress within a structure depends on how the structure functions and in which direction the center of pressure is moved. Bones and joints are stressed under compression and torsion. Compression becomes greater with increasing ground reaction force. Therefore, moving the center of pressure away from an area of damaged bone or joint should decrease the stress, further injury, and pain. Tendons and ligaments are stressed under tension. In the horse's foot, moving the center of pressure toward the tendon or ligament reduces the tension in the tendon and vice versa. As such, moving the center of pressure has the opposite effect on bones and joints, which are stressed under compression compared with its effects on tendons and ligaments, which are stressed under tension. Other soft tissue

Box 1
Definitions

Distribution of force

Anywhere there is contact between the body and the ground, there is a force between the body and the ground. However, the force is not necessarily evenly distributed. For example, if a horse is standing on sand, the pressure is primarily distributed across the middle of the foot, including the sole and part of the frog. However, if the horse is standing on a flat unyielding surface, most of the pressure is distributed around the perimeter of the foot at the interface of the ground and wall (**Fig. 1**).

Ground reaction force

The ground reaction force is the force exerted by the ground on a body that is in contact with the ground. It is represented as a vector that represents the sum of all individual forces on the surface of the body in consideration (**Fig. 2**).

Center of pressure

The center of pressure it that point through which the ground force acts. It is also called the point of zero moment because it is that point at which all the moments created by forces on the object, in this case the horse's foot, cancel out each other (**Fig. 3**).

Moment (torque)

A moment is the tendency of force to cause rotation about an axis. It is calculated as the product of the length of the moment arm and the component of the force that is at right angles to the lever arm. If there are 2 equal, but opposite, moments acting around an axis, no movement occurs (see **Fig. 3**).

Viscoelasticity

Viscoelasticity is a property of a material that describes the way it responds to the application of force in relation to time. It demonstrates both elastic and viscous behavior. Elastic objects, such as a metal spring, deform immediately when subject to a linear stress and return to prior length immediately the stress is removed. Viscous materials, such as honey, resist linear shear and strain when subject to stress but do not return to normal when the stress is removed. As such, a viscoelastic object responds differently if a force is applied to it surface rapidly compared with a force that is applied gradually. Rapid application of force elicits elastic behavior in which the object deforms but rapidly returns to its original shape. Application of force over an extended time period causes the object to deform gradually, and when the force is removed, the object gradually returns to its normal shape. Many biologic materials behave in a viscoleastic manner, and the hoof wall, when subject to stress, behaves similarly.

structures in the foot to be considered are the lamellae and solar dermis. The lamellae are most likely to suffer mechanical injury when under excessive tension (though compression might perhaps cause other damage such as ischemia). However, in contrast to ligaments and tendons, moving the center of pressure to one side of the foot increases the tension/shear stress in the lamellae on that side of the foot. Compression of the solar corium potentially causes bruising at whichever point the pressure is increased.

The center or pressure can be deliberately moved in the frontal plane by physically increasing the length of one side of the foot relative to the other (**Fig. 4**).[4,5] The length of one side of the foot can be increased by trimming and/or with shoeing. Increasing the length of the wall with shoeing is most frequently done by inserting a pad between the shoe and the hoof capsule. Additionally, a shoe with either branch with a thicker web than the other increases the length of one side of the foot. The length of one side of the foot can be functionally lengthened by any farriery manipulation that causes one side of the shoe to descend into a soft substrate more than the other side (see distribution

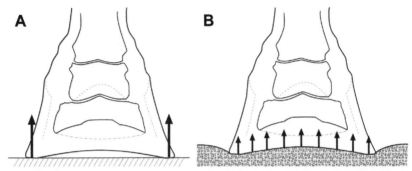

Fig. 1. When a foot is standing on a flat firm surface, the area of contact is primarily the perimeter of the ground surface of hoof, and hence this is the area over which the force of weight bearing is distributed (*A*). When the same foot is on a soft surface that deforms readily, then the same force is distributed over the ground surface of the foot (*B*). (*Courtesy of* Andrew Parks, VetMB, MS, MRCVS, University of Georgia, Athens, GA.)

of pressure). This can be accomplished by increasing the ground surface contact area of one side of the foot compared with the other. This is achieved by changing the relative widths of the web, adding a bar or heel plate, or using a partial pour-in pad. Alternatively, the functional length of one side of the foot may be increased by creating a medial or lateral extension with the shoe (see extensions below) because the extension creates greater leverage about the anatomic center of the foot when the horse is standing on soft ground; however, while the author has used this maneuver to good effect on occasion, the concept is based on theoretical reasoning rather than scientific observation.

Distribution of Force on the Ground Surface of the Foot

The distribution of force may be changed to increase/decrease weight bearing by one area of the foot to reduce/increase weight bearing by another part of the foot. Altering

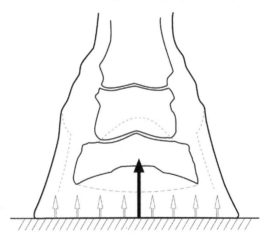

Fig. 2. The ground reaction force is force exerted by the ground on a body that is in contact with it. The force is distributed variably over the area of contact, but represented by a single vector; as a vector it has a direction and magnitude. Additionally, the force has a point of action referred to as the center of pressure. (*Courtesy of* Andrew Parks, VetMB, MS, MRCVS, University of Georgia, Athens, GA.)

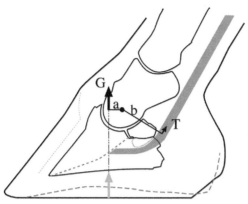

Fig. 3. The distal interphalangeal joint is a ginglymus joint, and as such it is capable of flexion or extension. When the horse is standing at rest, the foot is stationary in relation to the ground. The tendency for a body to rotate about an axis is related to the net moments about the joint; the extensor moment is the product of the ground reaction force (*G*) and the length of the extensor moment arm (*a*), and the flexor moment is the product of the force in the deep flexor tendon (*T*) and the length of the flexor moment arm (*b*). Therefore, at rest the flexor moment (*G* × *a*) is equal to the extensor moment (*T* × *b*). (*Courtesy of Andrew Parks, VetMB, MS, MRCVS, University of Georgia, Athens, GA.*)

the distribution of force across the ground surface of the foot cannot be done without regard to the center of pressure. If the distribution is done in a functionally symmetrically manner about the center of pressure, the center of pressure will not change; that is, it is possible to reduce or increase or decrease overall area of contact between the foot and the ground without altering the center of pressure. However, if done in a functionally asymmetrical manner, it will cause a concurrent change in the center of pressure.

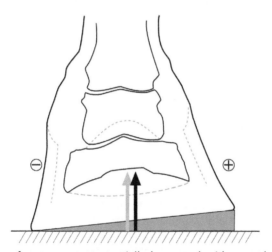

Fig. 4. The center of pressure can potentially be moved with several different farriery maneuvers. In this example, a wedge is applied transversely across the foot so that one side of the limb is effectively lengthened in relation to the other. This causes the center of pressure to move toward the elongated side. Consequently, the compressive stresses are increased in the lengthened side and decreased in the contralateral side. (*Courtesy of Andrew Parks, VetMB, MS, MRCVS, University of Georgia, Athens, GA.*)

Given that a horse that is shod in a standard fashion standing on a firm surface bears weight primarily on the wall and the immediately adjacent sole, recruiting additional ground surface for weight bearing involves weight bearing by either additional sole, frog, or bars or a combination of the three. Of course, on softer surfaces into which the shoe can descend, these additional areas may already be bearing some weight. The role of the sole, frog, and bars in normal weight bearing and transmission of the ground reaction force to the skeletal structures of the digit is only partially understood. It is known that for a traditionally shod horse standing on firm ground, the pressure is distributed around the periphery of the foot.[6] It is also known that for a horse that has been allowed to go bare foot and then stands on a deformable surface like sand, the pressure is largely distributed across the center of the foot including the sole and frog.[6] The combination of this evidence suggests that at least under some circumstances almost any part of the ground surface of the foot can withstand the load associated with weight bearing.

However, it does not describe how the load is transferred from the ground surface of the foot to the distal phalanx. While it might intuitively seem that when the load is distributed across a broad band from quarter to quarter, the weight is transferred from the sole directly to the distal phalanx, finite element analysis suggests that the forces associated with weight bearing are transmitted through the substance of the sole to the wall, and thus through the lamellae to the distal phalanx.[7] The significance for farriery is in how the ground surface of the foot can be loaded therapeutically. While a healthy thick sole is capable of being the primary loading surface of the hoof capsule, regardless of the mechanism by which the load is transferred to the distal phalanx, with reduced thickness, the normal function of the sole becomes impaired. Additionally, finite element analysis indicates that as the foot expands, the sole descends.[7] Therefore, any farriery manipulation that limits descent of the sole may also limit expansion of the foot at the quarters, an event that is associated with damping impact vibrations.

Redistributing the force across the ground surface of a horse's foot is used in shod horses to recruit weight bearing by part or all of the ground surface of the hoof capsule between the branches of the shoe to decrease weight bearing by the adjacent wall. For example, in horses with laminitis, the ground surface of the foot is frequently recruited to bear weight to decrease weight bearing by the wall. The angles of the sole, bars, and frog may be recruited to bear weight to decrease weight bearing by the wall at the heels in horses with underrun heels. There are, of course, limitations to both these techniques. In horses with laminitis, loading the sole may create sufficient pressure to cause pain, and in horses with underrun heels, the angle of the sole, bar, and frog may be sufficiently distorted or traumatized to limit their role in weight bearing. Clearly, when only part of the ground surface is recruited to bear weight, it is also very likely to cause the center of pressure to move.

Motion About the Distal Interphalangeal Joint

One of the goals of therapeutic shoeing is to decrease the stresses in structures on the flexor surface of the distal interphalangeal joint during the latter half of the stride, particularly just before breakover. During this phase of the stride, the accessory ligament of the deep digital flexor tendon and the tendon distal to the insertion of the accessory ligament are under the greatest tension,[8] as are the suspensory and distal sesamoidean ligaments of the navicular bone. The navicular bone is also under compressive stress from the tension in the deep digital flexor tendon.[9] There are 2 recognized techniques to decrease these stresses: moving the point of breakover in a palmar direction and elevating the heels.

Moving the point of breakover in a palmar direction has been shown to decrease the length of the moment arm about the distal interphalangeal joint at the moment of breakover (**Fig. 5**).[10] Additionally, it may cause breakover to occur slightly earlier in the stride at a higher ground reaction force,[11] but it does not significantly reduce the duration of breakover.[10,12,13] Furthermore, it does not change the maximum compressive force on the navicular bone.[10] The principal benefits of moving the point of breakover in a palmar direction may be that it smoothens hoof unrollment (**Fig. 6**)[13] and causes breakover to occur slightly earlier.

Elevating the heels shortens the moment arm of the extensor moment because it causes the center of pressure to move toward the center of rotation (**Fig. 7**). Therefore, given no change in the ground reaction force, there is a decrease in the maximal extensor moment.[9] For the foot to maintain its stable position on the ground, there must be a corresponding decrease in the flexor moment, which is associated with a decrease in the strain in the deep digital flexor tendon[14] because the flexor moment arm is constant when the foot is flat on the ground. The decrease in the strain in the deep digital flexor tendon and the reduction in the angle of the deep digital flexor tendon about the navicular bone decrease maximum pressure on the navicular bone.[9] However, heel elevation does not cause the heels to be unloaded and causes a delay in the dorsal movement of the center of pressure at breakover.[5,11] Additionally, elevating the heels beyond a straight foot-pastern axis causes a potentially deleterious redistribution of pressure dorsal within the distal interphalangeal joint and increases distal interphalangeal joint pressure.[15]

Traction

Altering the traction provided by a shoe is primarily a performance enhancer, and in doing so it may reduce the risk of injury, but it is only occasionally used as a direct therapeutic measure. Traction is determined by friction between the ground and the foot. This is in part related to the materials and contours of the opposing surfaces. In large part the ground surface is predetermined. Plastic shoes may reduce slippage on a concrete surface and studs reduce slippage on grass.[16,17]

Movement of the Foot During the Flight Phase of the Stride

The flight phase of the stride has received attention for 2 principal reasons: animation of gait of show and performance horses and correction of between-limb interference. Of these, only the latter is used therapeutically. The correction of between-limb

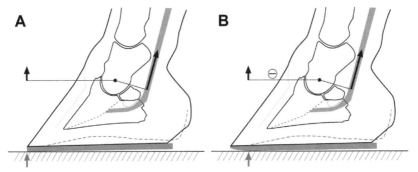

Fig. 5. At beginning of breakover (ie, the minute the heels leave the ground), the center of pressure is at the toe (*A*). By moving the point of breakover in a palmar direction by rolling the toe, the length of the moment arm at breakover is reduced (*B*). (*Courtesy of* Andrew Parks, VetMB, MS, MRCVS, University of Georgia, Athens, GA.)

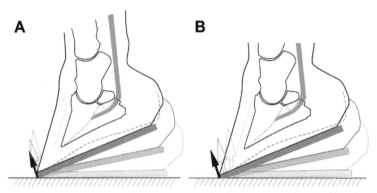

Fig. 6. As the foot rotates about the toe between the beginning and end of breakover, with a regular toe the pivot point stays the same (*A*). If the toe is rolled (or rockered), then the point about which the foot pivots changes as the foot unrolls (*B*). (*Courtesy of* Andrew Parks, VetMB, MS, MRCVS, University of Georgia, Athens, GA.)

interference primarily focuses on the interdependence between the flight and the stance phases of the stride and to a lesser extent on the animation of the gait. The manner in which a horse breaks over may influence the way the distal limb moves during protraction and the way the foot contacts the ground influences the way the foot is positioned on the ground. Therefore, these manipulations are directed at either changing the way the foot breaks over, typically to speed up the front feet or slow down the hind feet, and alter the way the foot is positioned as it lands. There is little information available on the effects of these manipulations. One study examined the effect of changing the angulation of hind feet by selective trimming to lengthen the toe of the hind feet in relation to the heels; this resulted in a tendency toward a delayed breakover and increasing breakover time, but normal coordination was restored during the swing phase of the stride so that the timing of impact was not affected.[18]

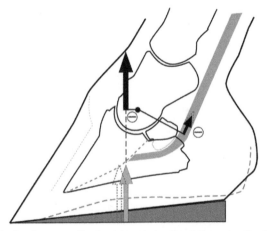

Fig. 7. Elevating the heels causes the foot to rotate about the axis of rotation of the distal interphalangeal joint in the direction of flexion. This is associated with a decrease in the tension in the deep digital flexor tendon and a shortening of the extensor moment arm. (*Courtesy of* Andrew Parks, VetMB, MS, MRCVS, University of Georgia, Athens, GA.)

Another study demonstrated that increasing the length of the toe of forefeet increased the duration of breakover.[19]

THE ANATOMY AND FUNCTION OF THE SHOE

In its most simple form, a horse shoe is a rectangular bar of metal curved to fit the outer margin of the ground surface of the hoof wall that is sufficiently wide to cover the distal wall and a small amount of the adjacent sole, and then punched to accept nails for attachment of the shoe to the foot. At the mid quarter, the shoe should be fit flush with the outer edge of the hoof wall and then gradually extended 2 to 3 mm abaxially as it approaches the heels to accommodate expansion of the foot and 3 to 4 mm caudally to anticipate forward movement of the shoe in relation to the heels as the hoof grows.

Changing Cross-Sectional Profile of the Branches of the Shoe

There are 3 main modifications that may be made to the cross-sectional profile of a horse shoe: change the width or depth of the web, change the profile of the rims, and add creases. With these different manipulations, it is possible to alter the distribution of force, change the center of pressure, and change the motion about the distal interphalangeal joint.

The most common modifications to the basic shoe pattern involve modifications of the ground surface and the inner and outer rims. If the most basic shoe pattern is that of a flat shoe punched to accept nails, the simplest modification is to alter the width or depth of the shoe. Increasing the width of a shoe increases the surface area of the ground surface of the shoe and would therefore be expected to decrease traction, a technique applied on the hind feet of reining horses to increase their ability to slide. Conversely, decreasing the width of the shoe is likely to increase traction, primarily on a ground surface that yields. If the width of the web is changed nonsymmetrically, it will cause the area with a wider web to descend into a soft surface more than that with a narrower web, thus moving the center of pressure toward that area that descends into the surface least. Similarly, if the web is thicker on one side of the shoe than the other then the center of pressure will move toward the side of the shoe with the thicker branch, even on a flat unyielding ground surface.

From the perspective of therapeutic farriery, the most important modifications affecting the rims of the shoe are treatments that are performed at the toe, specifically rounding or rockering the toe. These both change the length of the moment arm at the beginning of breakover. Squaring the toe, although not strictly the same, may achieve a similar effect. Beveling the outer rim around the full circumference of the shoe will reduce the moment arm about the distal interphalangeal joint when the horse breaks over toward one side of the foot or the other.

The addition of a crease to a shoe is done to increase traction, presumably by adding 2 edges that may enhance the gripping of a deformable surface. Additionally, the crease may fill with dirt that would have a greater coefficient of friction than steel on the ground. Creases may encompass part or the entire circumference of the shoe. For general traction they are used around the full length of the shoe. In general, creases are primarily used as a performance-enhancing measure. However, creases may be selectively applied at the toe for traction during breakover or on one branch of the shoe when the intent is to delay breakover of one side of the shoe.

In addition to modifications made to the ground surface of the shoe, the foot surface of a wide web shoe may be seated out to relieve pressure on the sole of flat-footed horses.

Bars

A bar is any part of the shoe that extends from one branch to the other. There are 4 most commonly applied types of bar shoe: straight bar shoe, egg-bar shoe, heart bar shoe, and egg-bar heart bar shoe (also called a full support shoe). Because all these shoes extend from one heel to the other, they increase the area of ground contact of the palmar aspect of the shoe. By increasing the palmar ground contact, they may cause a change in the distribution of force and cause the center of pressure to move in a palmar direction when a horse is working on a soft ground surface. How much they cause a shift in the center of pressure is related to how much they increase the surface area and how far removed from the center of pressure is this increased surface area. Therefore, an egg-bar heart bar shoe would be expected to have a greater effect than a straight bar shoe, with the other 2 types of shoe having an intermediate effect.

Bars may also protect an underlying structure from direct pressure from the ground. They are also used to stabilize the 2 branches of the shoe; the effectiveness of this is open to question, but it is more likely to be effective when the shoes are made of aluminum. Bar shoes are commonly used in this manner when a portion of the hoof wall has been resected or used in conjunction with side clips for horses with distal phalanx fractures.

Pads

Pads are a layer of leather or synthetic material that is interposed between the shoe and the hoof. The pad may cover the entire ground surface of the foot or just part of it. Additionally, they may be flat or wedged. Complete pads cover the entire ground surface of the foot. The most common type of partial pad is the rim pad, which is cut to mimic the shape of the shoe and leaves the majority of the sole and frog exposed; however, partial pads can be designed to cover any particular part of the ground surface of the foot as desired.

Pads may be used to prevent the sole from coming into direct contact with the ground, to provide damping of impact vibrations, change the ground surface distribution of force, and change the center of pressure. Viscoelastic pads, be they partial or complete, are able to dampen the vibrations associated with impact. Unfortunately, it is not always possible to tell which commercial pads behave in this way. Pads that extend into the space between the branches of the shoe may increase ground contact in a specific part of the ground surface of the foot; for example, there are pads formed to mimic the action of a heart bar shoe. Pads that are in the form of a wedge can alter dorsopalmar or mediolateral balance and, in doing so, change the location of the center of pressure and change which part of the foot makes first contact with the ground.

Pads are commonly used to protect the sole, though it has been argued that by lowering the surface that contacts the ground between the branches of the shoe, they may actually increase trauma under some circumstances. Rim pads lift the sole farther from the ground; however, it may also allow the sole or frog to descend excessively if they are structurally impaired and/or inadequately supported by the adjacent or underlying structures.

There is one category of pad that is not a true pad in the traditional sense of the word that needs separate consideration—the pour-in-pad. Pour-in-pads are formed by dispensing a liquid polymer into the space between the branches of the shoe, the cup of the sole, and the sulci of the frog, which then hardens in situ. These materials solidify to various degrees of hardness. As an alternative to the liquid polymers, 2-part silicone putty may be used. How well these different pads function depends on the rigidity of the poured in material and the thickness of the sole; thick soles may tolerate a rigid pad and very thin soles may not tolerate a pour-in-pad at all. These pads are used to redistribute weight bearing away from the walls. If used as partial pads, they can redirect weight bearing locally; this is frequently done in the palmar half of the foot to increase weight bearing by the frog, bars, and angles of the sole to either decrease the amount the palmar half of the foot descends into the substrate or reduce weight bearing by the walls at the heels.

The cavity underneath full pads is packed; traditionally, the space under leather pads is packed with pine tar and oakum and the space under plastic pads with silicone, but other synthetic and natural products have been substituted. Thrush is a potential sequel following application of full pads because of the moisture trapped underneath them, particularly if the frog is unhealthy to start with. Some materials are better than others at preventing thrush from developing.

Extensions

The term "extension" applies to any part of a shoe that extends past the perimeter of a normal shoe that makes contact with the ground; a normal shoe extends beyond the perimeter of the foot just enough to allow for growth of the foot between shoeings and expansion of the heels. An extension may be placed at any point around the perimeter of the foot, though typically they are used on the dorsal surface, palmar surface, or lateral surface and in foals with angular limb deformities on the medial surface. Their function depends on the surface on which the horse is standing or moving and where they are placed around the circumference of the shoe. In general terms, they may be used to change the center of pressure and influence motion about the distal interphalangeal joint.

On a yielding ground surface, extensions decrease the tendency of the side of the shoe with the extension to drop into the substrate compared with the rest of the shoe; as such, they function as wedges and shift the center of pressure toward the side of the extension. When a horse is in motion, any extension that causes that part of the shoe to contact the ground earlier than the shoe would otherwise will alter the way the foot lands. For example, a lateral heel extension (trailer) that causes the lateral heel to contact the ground sooner than normal will cause the foot to rotate to that side as it lands. Similarly, an extension positioned around the perimeter of the dorsal third of the foot is likely to prolong contact with the ground at that point at the end of the stance phase of the stride, thus altering the way the foot rotates as it lifts off, and potentially changing the point of breakover in the process.

Extensions can be formed in several ways. The simplest to comprehend is that created by welding a piece of metal to the outside rim of the shoe at any point around its perimeter, though the same result can be achieved through forging. However, a medial or lateral extension can be created just as easily by spreading the branches of the shoe and re-punching one branch coarsely, so that when applied, the re-punched branch extends farther beyond the perimeter of the foot on that side. Heel extensions include any lengthening of the branches of the shoe in a palmar direction or inclusion of an egg bar in the shoe. Short straight extensions are sometimes applied to both branches of hind shoe worn by horses in work. A longer, abaxially angled extension is sometimes applied to the lateral branch of a hind shoe.

Traction Devices

Traction devices for the purpose of this discussion are any device that is added to the ground surface of the shoe with the goal of increasing friction between the shoe and the ground. They have limited use in therapeutic farriery. As such, they are usually used to reduce interference between limbs in standardbred horses, either by turning the foot as it lands or delaying breakover of one side of the shoe in relation to the other. How this is done is very much up to the experience of the individual.

APPLICATION OF PRINCIPLES TO DISEASE

To apply the goals of farriery to any given disease, it is important to know which structures are injured and how altering the stresses on those structures will either reduce pain or improve function. In general, bones and articular surfaces are likely to be damaged by excessive compression, whereas tendons and ligaments are damaged when they are under excessive tension. The lamellae would also be expected to be injured under excessive tension. Compression of bones and joints can be reduced by moving the stresses away from the affected area. Conversely, the tension in tendons and ligaments is reduced by moving the center or pressure toward the affected structure. Damaged lamellae are protected by moving the center of pressure away from the part of the foot with the damage.

It should be emphasized that, to the author's knowledge, all the farriery manipulations described next to improve foot function with different diseases are based on theoretical reasoning or individual clinician experience: these are not case-control evidence-derived practices. The following is not a complete list of solutions but rather contains examples of how to think about using farriery to treat these select diseases. The principles can be extrapolated to other circumstances as they are encountered.

Laminitis

Pertinent pathophysiology
Therapeutic farriery is the mainstay for treating horses with chronic unstable laminitis. The lamellae are the primary tissue affected, and they are most painful and subject to further injury when loaded excessively in relation to the damage they have sustained. Additionally, because the distal phalanx displaces, it compresses the soft tissues in the dorsal part of the sole that makes weight bearing by the dorsal sole painful. The disease is complicated because the lamellae may break down at any point around the perimeter of the hoof from heel to heel. Before displacement, there is currently no practical method of imaging to determine where the greatest damage may be, and response to hoof testers or different supporting devices is the best way to infer where the injury is most severe.

Goals

a. To move the center of pressure away from the most damaged lamellae (with dorsal rotation, this involves decreasing the tension in the deep digital flexor tendon).
b. To redistribute pressure away from the lamellae.
c. To avoid/reduce pressure on sensitive areas of the sole.
d. To facilitate breakover.

Implementation

a. The most effective way to move the center pressure is to apply a wedge on the side of the foot opposite to the damaged lamellae. For example, if the dorsal lamellae are injured and the horse has dorsal capsular and phalangeal rotation, heel elevation would move the center of pressure toward the center of rotation of the distal interphalangeal joint and, in doing so, decreases the tension in the deep digital flexor tendon. For horses with unilateral distal displacement, a wedge applied to the healthier side of the foot would move the center of pressure away from the most damaged lamellae. However, the author prefers extending the shoe on the same side that would have had a wedge, which will have a similar but milder effect if the horse is standing on a soft substrate.

b. Redistributing pressure away from the lamellae is attempted by recruiting parts of the ground surface of the foot to bear weight (without impacting goal "c").

c. Limiting pressure can be achieved by ensuring no contact of the sensitive part of the foot by the ground or the shoe. Application of a shoe will elevate the foot from the ground. The shoe may require seating out to limit pressure on the adjacent sole.

d. The moment arm at breakover can be reduced in many ways: rolling/rockering the toe, squaring the toe, setting the shoe back, or using an open-toed shoe. Many shoes including heart bar, egg bar, open-toed shoes, 4-point rail shoes/Equine Digital Support System (Equine Digital Support System, Inc., Penrose, CO, USA), and wooden shoes have been used to attain some or all of these goals. Because experience with one or two leads to the greatest likelihood of success, most clinicians favor 1 or 2 techniques; for this reason the author has the most experience with the 4-point rail shoe/EDSS and, to a lesser extent, wooden shoes and egg bar shoes, and not because the alternatives are necessarily less effective. Each shoe must be judged on its own merits as to how it can achieve the above stated goals.

Collateral Ligament Injury

Pertinent pathophysiology

The collateral ligament is injured from excessive strain, either repetitive lower-grade strain or an abrupt high-level strain, and following injury, any aspect of weight bearing or movement that imposes marked strain on the ligament will cause pain and/or impede healing. Therefore, farriery measures employed should attempt to limit the lengthening of the ligament at rest or during motion.

Goals

a. Move the center of pressure toward the side of the affected collateral ligament.

b. Ease the torque about the distal interphalangeal joint when turning away from the affected side.

Implementation

a. Any manipulation that increases the surface area of ground contact on one side of the foot compared with the other will shift the center of pressure to that side if a horse is standing on a yielding surface. The farther from the median plane of the limb is the increased surface area, the greater effect it will have. Increasing the width of the branch of the shoe on the affected side, narrowing the branch of the opposite branch, and/or extending the ground contact abaxially may all accomplish this goal if the horse is standing on a yielding substrate (though the latter is less likely to be used on the medial side of the foot). While a wedge to elevate the affected side of the foot will achieve the same effect on soft or hard surface, it is a more aggressive maneuver so the unintended consequences are likely to be greater, and the author has not seen it used.

b. This can be achieved by rounding the outer rim of the opposite branch of the shoe.

Imbalance

Pertinent pathophysiology

A satisfying description of balance and imbalance and that meets everyone's needs remains elusive. The author considers balance to be cover both the relationship between the hoof capsule and the underlying phalanges and the relationship between the hoof and the ground. Additionally, the concepts of conformation and balance are interrelated. For the purpose of this discussion, conformation will be considered to be the shape of the distal limb at rest excluding the hoof capsule.

The functional effect of prolonged imbalance is excessive stress at one place around the hoof capsule, frequently associated with reduced stress elsewhere that is manifest by reduction in growth rate of overstressed wall, development of capsular distortions such as flares or underruning, and movement of the coronary band in relation to the underlying phalanges.

Balance will be considered to be the shape of the hoof capsule and its relationship to the rest of the distal limb and the ground; this can be summarized as optimal manner of landing/breakover and weight bearing during the stance phase of the stride. Clearly, they are interrelated but worth separating because of the therapeutic approach needed. Poor conformation in an adult cannot be corrected because the underlying determinant of the shape of the distal limb is the shape and arrangement of the bones, though it can be compensated for. In contrast, poor balance may be improved, if not corrected; this is because the hoof is continuously growing and can readily change shape. Imbalance is complicated because there are immediate effects of changing the shape of the hoof due to its viscoelastic nature and chronic effects that result from altered hoof growth and distortion of the capsule beyond that of visco-elastic changes. Poor conformation or balance is not a disease in itself but may predispose to other diseases/injuries, though documentation of this is poor. Imbalance that is not a consequence of poor conformation may well respond to trimming and allowing the horse to go barefoot because the absence of a shoe allows the hoof to wear naturally, allows the hoof capsule to move in relation to the distal phalanx more readily, and allows one part of the hoof to move in relation to another. However, when either this fails or the nature of athletic endeavor requires shoeing, the following measures may be employed.

Dorsopalmar imbalance
Goals
a. Restore a straight foot-pastern axis.

Implementation
a. If the foot-pastern axis is broken back, then damaged or underrun heels and excessive toe length must be addressed. This may provide satisfactory correction, but that is frequently not the case. If the horse does not need to be shod for exercise purposes, it may be advisable to leave the horse barefoot. Full correction of the axis may be achieved with a wedge pad, but this frequently reduces future healthy heel growth. Instead, providing ground surface contact with the frog, bars, and angles of the sole with a partial pour in pad or a heel plate with silicone putty may be a better option; even though it does not immediately correct the foot-pastern axis, it may provide a better opportunity for restoring the health of damaged heels.

Mediolateral imbalance
Goals
a. Restore optimal mediolateral distribution of weight bearing.

Implementation
a. It is always preferable to restore the optimal mediolateral weight bearing by trimming the foot if possible. However, when one wall is too short to permit appropriate

leveling of the ground surface, then the shorts side of the foot can be lengthened in several ways: using a shoe in which the branch on the shorter side of the hoof capsule is thicker that the opposite side, placing a shim between the shoe and the hoof on the short side of the capsule, or using a composite to extend the length of the wall on the shorter side.

Navicular Syndrome

Pertinent pathophysiology
Navicular syndrome was initially so called because, in addition to the bone itself, many of the structures surrounding the navicular bone are likely to be injured under similar circumstances; this has subsequently been confirmed with magnetic resonance imaging. The biomechanics of the phases of the stride indicate that the tension in the deep digital flexor tendon and pressure on the navicular bone are greatest during the end of the support phase of the stride and the beginning of breakover, suggesting that this is the point in the stride most likely to be associated with pain secondary to disease of the navicular apparatus. Additionally, the vibrations associated with initial impact have also been implicated.

Goals

a. Decrease the tension in the deep digital flexor tendon at breakover.
b. Make the process of breaking over smoother.
c. Decrease tension in the deep digital flexor tendon during the stance phase of the stride.
d. Decrease impact vibrations at the beginning of the stance phase of the stride.

Implementation

a, b. These 2 goals may be addressed simultaneously. Any of the mechanisms that move the point of breakover in a palmar direction will shorten the moment arm at breakover. However, it appears that those manipulations that involve a marked rounding of the surface of the toe, so that the foot unrolls over an extended surface rather than about a single point offers the advantage that is smoothes out the process and may make transitions in tension in internal structures more gradual.

c. Any manipulation that causes the distal interphalangeal joint to be less extended during the support phase of the stride will decrease the tension in the deep flexor tendon at the same time. For a horse that is exercising on a soft substrate, this can be achieved by using a shoe with a straight bar shoe; alternatively, an egg bar shoe will do the same more aggressively. These both work by decreasing the tendency of the palmar aspect of the shoe to descend into a yielding substrate. A wedge pad will decrease extension of the distal interphalangeal joint on any surface. The least aggressive of these that accomplishes the goals is advisable.

d. A combination of energy absorbing pads and synthetic shoes may decrease the frequency and magnitude of impact vibrations.

Pedal Osteitis

Pertinent pathophysiology
Pedal osteitis is a radiographic symptom that is thought to be related to chronic inflammation of the subsolar tissues adjacent to the margins of the distal phalanx. As such, the most likely cause is trauma to the sole, particularly bruising. Therefore, the principal inciting cause of pain is pressure on the sole, from either prolonged low-grade ground or shoe contact, or transient higher impacts. As such, it is more

likely to occur in horses with flat soles. It would be logical to expect impact vibrations to cause pain if there is inflammation between the sole and the distal phalanx.

Goals

a. Limit contact with the outer margins of the sole with shoe and/or ground; in essence, the pressure is on the outer margins of the sole and redistributed to the wall.
b. Decrease impact vibrations at the beginning of the stance phase of the stride.

Implementation

a. Any shoe lifts the sole off the ground to decrease ground contact, but the shoe itself may cause undue pressure on the periphery of the sole. This can be reduced/avoided by seating out the hoof surface of the shoe. The use of full pads for pedal osteitis has also been advocated because the pad will cause some dissipation of the force of impact; however, their use has been questioned because the pad covers the concavity of the sole, and therefore presents a surface that is closer to the ground and more likely to be impacted by an irregular ground surface than if no pad were present.
b. Reduction of concussion associated with impact is accomplished as previously described.

Degenerative Joint Disease of the Interphalangeal Joints

Degenerative joint disease is an irreversible process that is associated with a decrease in the integrity of the surface of the articular cartilage and reduction in the range of motion. Pain is caused by concussion and excessive flexion or extension/dorsiflexion.

Goals

a. Facilitate ease of movement by reducing the lever arm at the point of breakover (at the toe in forward motion and at the toe quarter junction when the horse is turning).
b. Limit concussion associated with impact.

Implementation

a. Any of the common techniques to reduce the length of the lever arm at the toe of the shoe may be employed. However, for horses with interphalangeal degenerative joint disease, it is also commonly recommended to aggressively roll all around the perimeter of the shoe as well; this type of shoe is called a roller motion shoe (note: this term is used inconsistently is sometimes applied to other types of shoe).
b. Reduction of concussion associated with impact is accomplished as previously described.

SUMMARY

Our knowledge has improved significantly over the last 25 years, and the range of tools and devices at our disposal has increased even more. With all this available, it is easy for a clinician to fall into a trap when venturing into therapeutic farriery; that is, the search for the perfect appliance/combination of appliances that, once found, will resolve any horse's problems. Unfortunately, while there are some horses that can be markedly improved and some that can be partially helped, there are always horses for which therapeutic farriery will be of no benefit. The skill is in recognizing which category a horse falls into, and then understanding the principles and mastering the techniques to improve them when possible. For the newcomer it should be some consolation to know that even the most experienced clinicians are constantly learning because there is so much that we all have yet to discover. It must be remembered that in the course of trial and error, errors of judgment are a necessary part of learning what is best for a horse; just try to recognize and avoid repeating them.

REFERENCES

1. Benoit P, Barrey E, Regnault JC, et al. Comparison of the damping effect of different shoeing by the measurement of hoof acceleration. Acta Anat (Basel) 1993;146(2–3):109–13.
2. Dyhre-Poulsen P, Smedegaard HH, Roed J, et al. Equine hoof function investigated by pressure transducers inside the hoof and accelerometers mounted on the first phalanx. Equine Vet J 1994;26(5):362–6.
3. Back W. Synthetic shoes attenuate hoof impact in the trotting warmblood horse. Equine Comp Exerc Physiol 2006;3:143–55.
4. Colahan P, Leach D. Center of pressure location of the hoof with and without hoof wedges. Equine Exerc Physiol 1991;3:113–9.
5. Wilson AM, Seelig TJ, Shield RA, et al. The effect of foot imbalance on point of force application in the horse. Equine Vet J 1998;30(6):540–5.
6. Hood D, Taylor D, Wagner I. Effects of ground surface deformability, trimming, and shoeing on quasistatic hoof loading patterns in horses. Am J Vet Res 2001;62(6):895–900.
7. Davies H, Merritt J, Thomason J. Biomechanics of the equine foot. In: Floyd A, Mansmann R, editors. Equine podiatry. St Louis (MO): Elsevier; 2007. p. 42–56.
8. Meershoek LS, Lanovaz JL, Schamhardt HC, et al. Calculated forelimb flexor tendon forces in horses with experimentally induced superficial digital flexor tendinitis and the effects of application of heel wedges. Am J Vet Res 2002; 63(3):432–7.
9. Willemen MA, Savelberg HH, Barneveld A. The effect of orthopaedic shoeing on the force exerted by the deep digital flexor tendon on the navicular bone in horses. Equine Vet J 1999;31(1):25–30.
10. Eliashar E, McGuigan M, Rogers K, et al. A comparison of three horseshoeing styles on the kinetics of breakover in sound horses. Equine Vet J 2002;34(2):184–90.
11. Wilson A, McGuigan M. The biomechanical effect of wedged, eggbar, and extension shoes in sound and lame horses. Proc Am Assoc Equine Pract 2001;47: 339–43.
12. Clayton H, Sigafoos R. Effect of three shoe types on the duration of breakover in sound trotting horses. J Equine Vet Sci 1991;11:129–32.
13. van Heel MC, van Weeren PR, Back W. Shoeing sound warmblood horses with a rolled toe optimises hoof-unrollment and lowers peak loading during breakover. Equine Vet J 2006;38(3):258–62.
14. Lochner FK, Milne DW, Mills EJ, et al. In vivo and in vitro measurement of tendon strain in the horse. Am J Vet Res 1980;41(12):1929–37.
15. Viitanen MJ, Wilson AM, McGuigan HR, et al. Effect of foot balance on the intra-articular pressure in the distal interphalangeal joint in vitro. Equine Vet J 2003; 35(2):184–9.
16. Pardoe CH, Wilson AM. In vitro mechanical properties of different equine hoof wall crack fixation techniques. Equine Vet J 1999;31(6):506–9.
17. Harvey AM, Williams SB, Singer ER. The effect of lateral heel studs on the kinematics of the equine digit while cantering on grass. Vet J 2012;192(2):217–21.

18. Clayton HM. The effect of an acute hoof wall angulation on the stride kinematics of trotting horses. Equine Vet J Suppl 1990;9:86–90.
19. Balch O, Clayton H, Lanovaz J. Weight- and length-induced changes in limb kinematics in trotting horses. Am Assoc Equine Pract 1996;42:218–9.

Farriery for the Hoof with Low or Underrun Heels

Robert J. Hunt, DVM, MS

KEYWORDS

- Hoof • Hoof conformation • Underrun heels • Hoof angle
- Horn tubule curvature (collapse)

KEY POINTS

- Underrun heels, the most commonly encountered hoof abnormality, are a hoof condition in which the hoof angle measured at the heel is greater than 5° lower than the hoof angle measured at the toe.
- Underrun heels occur in a multitude of breeds and occupations; however, they are seen most commonly in the training and racing thoroughbred.
- After physical examination, radiographic evaluation of the foot is a particularly useful adjunct and provides information pertinent to the development of an appropriate treatment plan.
- There exists a great deal of controversy among farriers and veterinarians regarding proper treatment of underrun heels, which suggests that there is no single best way to manage the condition.
- Long-term, conscientious hoof care is mandatory for re-establishing normal form and function of the foot to maintain long-term soundness.

INTRODUCTION

The palmar half of the foot plays a critical role not only in soundness but also in the health and maintenance of the horse as a whole. It is subject to almost incomprehensible external and internal biomechanical forces, which inherently predispose the palmar foot to injury. There has likely been more attention given to the foot over the past half century than any other structure of the musculoskeletal system. Vast strides have been made by veterinarians and farriers regarding knowledge of the biomechanics and the anatomy and the function of the palmar foot. Some primary functions of the palmar foot are to dissipate shock and to withstand a complex array of biomechanical forces applied to the capsule and the internal structures of the foot. One possible sequela of repetitive exposure to these loading forces is distortion of the

The author has nothing to disclose.
Hagyard Equine Medical Institute, 4250 Iron Works Pike, Lexington, KY 40511-8412, USA
E-mail address: rhunt@hagyard.com

hoof. Such conformational changes are common and often are not associated with lameness; however, distortion disorders are believed to predispose the foot to secondary problems, which may lead to injury and/or lameness. The abnormality most frequently observed is the long toe–low heel or underrun heel syndrome. The disorder occurs in a variety of stages and degrees. The long toe–low heel conformation initially often has normal or relatively normal mass of the foot and normal internal structures. Over time, deformation of the horn tubules in the forward direction occurs, along with a forward shift of the foot in conjunction with a reduction of mass in both the heel bulbs and the frog. Despite the advancements in knowledge that have occurred over the past 50 years, there is still tremendous controversy surrounding both maintenance and treatment of these and other palmar foot abnormalities and disorders.

FORM AND FUNCTION

To understand the development and treatment of hoof distortion, it is helpful to have a cursory review of the form and function of the heels. It is important to realize that application of a static model to such a dynamic structure may yield erroneous results, and furthermore, in this brief review, complex forces applied to the foot during accelerated and multidirectional travel are disregarded. This discussion is brief and addresses primarily those parameters that affect the development of palmar hoof distortion. A comprehensive review of the form and function of the hoof has recently been performed by Parks, at the 52nd annual convention of the American Association of Equine Practitioners.

Fundamentally, the stride has 2 primary phases: the suspension phase and the stance phase. The suspension phase involves movement of the limb off the ground, whereas during the stance phase, the limb is in contact with the ground. The stance phase is further subdivided into the contact, impact, stance, and breakover phases. How the foot contacts the ground is largely individualized depending on the conformation of the horse and the flight pattern of the limb. In general, most horses land lateral quarter, heel first, or flat-footed. The contact portion of the stance phase is followed by the impact portion of the stance phase. On initial impact the vertical ground reaction force is low; however, high-frequency vibrations occur that are believed a significant source of injury. After impact, there is maximal expansion of the foot occurs during the first part of the stance phase after the oscillations of impact have subsided. This is followed by contraction of the heels to the width of the pre-expansion dimension, which is further followed by the contraction of the heels to a diameter smaller than that at the point of contact as the center of pressure moves toward the toe during the last portion of this phase. The majority of the dampening of the vertical component of the ground reaction force occurs between the hoof and the distal phalanx during this portion of the stance phase. Therefore, expansion of the palmar half of the foot seems related to energy absorption from the vertical component of the ground reaction force. Controversy exists over whether or not there is increased pressure in the digital cushion and, if so, whether it arises from increased frog pressure or descent of the second phalanx toward the digital cushion. This increase in pressure in the digital cushion is believed the origin of the expansion of the palmar aspect of the hoof. This function may be compromised by any conformational or locomotor alteration, which decreases the ability of the palmar foot to absorb the shock associated with movement. Any resulting imbalance of the foot not only impairs this natural function of the palmar hoof but also predisposes the foot to distortional changes and subsequent stress-induced injuries.

THE UNDERRUN HEEL SYNDROME

The term, *underrun heels*, is defined as a hoof condition in which the hoof angle measured at the heel is greater than 5° lower than the hoof angle measured at the toe.[1–4] This distortion may be referred to by several other descriptors: underslung heels, run-under heels, collapsed heels, and long toe–low heel conformation. An affected hoof may be mildly or severely distorted, with severe distortion resulting in heel collapse due to bending and crushing of horn tubules (**Fig. 1**). The condition is the most commonly encountered hoof abnormality.[5,6] Underrun heels occur in training and performance horses in virtually all working breeds, are unusual in juveniles, and may or may not be associated with lameness. Lameness is generally secondary in nature and may arise only as the underrun heels become severe or other distortion problems occur. In one group of sound performance horses that were evaluated, underrun heels were present in 52% of animals examined.[7] In another group of horses with chronic heel pain, the prevalence of underrun heels was 77%,[1] whereas in a different group of horses that were lame without evidence of navicular disease, 72.8% had underrun heels.[8] Among a group of 90 racehorses that were necropsied, 97.2% had underrun heels, and the severity of the underrun heels was correlated to an increased risk of catastrophic suspensory apparatus failures.[9] In a separate study in which 95 thoroughbred racehorses were necropsied, horses with a 10° or greater difference between toe and heel angles were 6.75 times more likely to undergo suspensory apparatus failure.[10]

Underrun heels may be justifiably viewed as a syndrome due to the complexity of factors involved in distortion of the hoof capsule and structures within the foot, which are affected due to the alteration of heel angle. Although a direct effect of underrun heels causing mechanical overload was not demonstrated in one study of a group of 31 horses,[11] the biomechanical theory of navicular disease and palmar foot pain

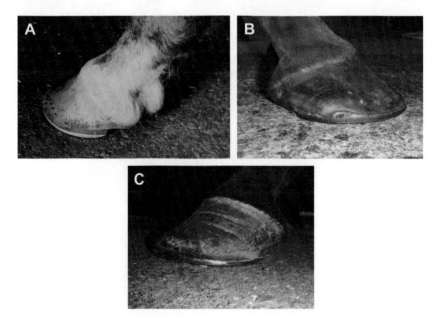

Fig. 1. (*A*) Moderately underrun heels, showing rolling forward of the horn tubules of the heel. Note the position of contact point of the heels. (*B*) An advanced case of underrun heels. (*C*) A moderate case of underrun heels.

suggests that abnormal forces are exerted on the navicular bone and its suspensory apparatus, resulting in degeneration of the bone. Deep digital flexor tendon tension plays an important role in the creation of this abnormal force. Horses with underrun heels tend to have increased compression of the navicular bone, associated with increased tensile forces on the deep digital flexor tendon.[12] Therefore, it is possible that underrun heels play a role in navicular syndrome.

Other pathologic conditions resulting from or occurring concomitantly with underrun heels include bruising, corns, abscessation, solar and wall separation, hoof cracks, bar cracks, sheared heels, atrophy or prolapsed of the digital cushion, subcapsular soft tissue injuries, and osteoarthritis of the distal interphalangeal joint (**Fig. 2**).[1,4,5,7,13] Documented evidence from multiple studies combined with clinical observation demonstrate that the underrun heel complex has a tremendous association with lameness and the potential for serious injury or death.

Underrun heels occur in a multitude of breeds and occupations; however, it is seen most commonly in the training and racing thoroughbred. Irrespective of the discipline or breed, the principles of therapy are in large part similar. The management of the hoof distortion may differ somewhat in show horses due to the extended length of the athletic career, the chronicity of the condition, the different loading forces placed on the foot during work, and the wider range of treatment devices available for use in treatment. Because the magnitude of the forces exerted on the foot varies with the speed, duration, and type of work, the development of more severe distortion and

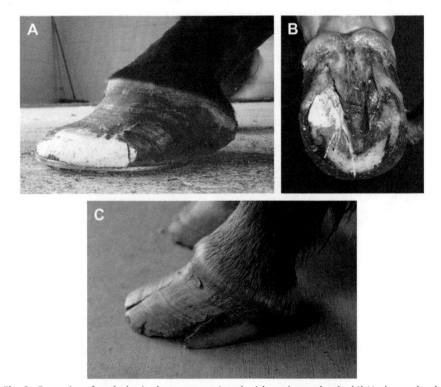

Fig. 2. Examples of pathologic changes associated with underrun heels. (*A*) Underrun heels with overgrown toe and distortion of dorsal hoof wall. (*B*) Example of deterioration and disease of the bars. (*C*) Underrun heels, diseased horn, and quarter crack.

a higher incidence of secondary problems within a shorter time period are more likely occurrences in racing thoroughbreds.

It is unusual for a juvenile thoroughbred racehorse to begin an athletic career with underrun heels although the potential for developing the condition may be recognizable during the weanling or yearling period. Manifestation of the distortion seems more an effect of workload than age. One characteristic that may predispose an animal to develop underrun heels is long, thin heels with an acute angle, compared with steep, thick short heels (Andrew Parks, MA, VetMB, MRCVS, DACVS, Athens, Georgia, and Mitch Taylor, CJF, Lexington, Kentucky, personal communication, June 2011). Conscientious trimming during this juvenile period is important and special attention should be given to heel structure and balance. The condition typically becomes more advanced and clinical problems develop with progression through training and racing. Presumably, while in intense exercise, the biomechanical forces applied to the hoof capsule have a tendency to pull the capsule in a dorsal direction during the load phase of the stride.[14] If the heels are in a weakened state and subjected to these forces, collapse and distortion is inevitable. In contrast, in racehorses that are undergoing rehabilitation and have decreased workloads, the underrun heels often improve; however, the distortion of the hoof tends to recur or worsen again once intense training resumes.[15,16]

ETIOLOGY

The underlying etiology and the pathogenesis of underrun heels are controversial. The most common supposition is that alteration of the hoof capsule originates at the toe, where the first level of distortion begins with shearing of dorsal lamellae created by downward toe force during stance phase of loading (dishing of the toe), which accompanies forward movement of the hoof wall relative to its original orientation with the distal phalanx. As a result of this dorsal movement of the wall, a dorsal shift of the heels occurs, which initiates tubular deformation.[17] Typically the first recognized clinical signs are a long toe and a low heel in conjunction with a weakening, thinning heel wall.[17] Another possible scenario that fosters the development of underrun heels begins at the heel region, in which there is primary deformation and collapse of the heels forward and axially. In these horses, frequently the tubular structure forward of the quarters is normal, and the foot pathology is more localized and restricted to the heel.

In both situations, a decline in the integrity of horn in the heel region is observed and is integral to the syndrome. Conformation changes in the heel on a macroscopic level begin with horn tubules curling in and compressing on themselves and showing no increase in heel height, followed by the characteristic bending forward of the horn tubules as they grow distally.[17] A forward shift of the hoof axis occurs, and weight-bearing surfaces shift forward, which places excessive stress on the structures on the palmar surface of the foot. Mechanical strength of the horn tubules declines as they grow forward, and potential subsequent bruising or tearing of the laminae of the region may occur.

As the condition advances, bending of the horn tubules may become extreme. Eventually the tubules may become parallel to the contact point of the ground and lose all ability to resist compression or absorb shock.[17] Collapse of the tubules is accompanied by progressive dorsal shifting of the hoof axis (**Fig. 3**). The contact point of the foot moves further forward, which perpetuates the tubule collapse and advances the distortion of the hoof. The tubular curvature may extend to the coronary band. These changes ultimately predispose the remaining palmar structures of the foot to overload, which, when combined with the low heel and dorsiflexion of the distal

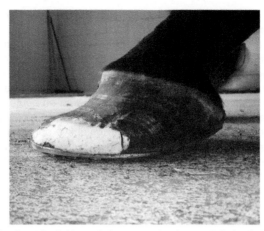

Fig. 3. Underrun heels with dishing of the toe and a forward shift of the hoof axis.

interphalangeal joint, create a negative angle between the solar surface of the distal phalanx and the ground (**Fig. 4**).[17] This dorsiflexion of the distal interphalangeal joint causes continued overloading of the heels and leads to a self-perpetuating cycle. As a result, there is an increased concentration of weight bearing on the palmar half of foot and increased strain on the deep digital flexor tendon. Secondarily, there may be insult to the circulation of the heel and soft tissue damage in this region, leading to the eventual reduction in soft tissue mass of the digital cushion or palmar prolapse of the digital cushion. These alterations may result in the loss of ability to dissipate energy of impact, which may further contribute to macroscopic conformational changes observed, including thinning of heels, wall separation, rolling in of heels axially, and compromise of the bars.

It has been suggested that there is a strong genetic basis to the syndrome based on the high incidence in racehorses.[18] At this date, genetic predisposition to underrun heels has not been proved or refuted; however, experience suggests that general hoof conformation and integrity may be largely influenced by pedigree. Thus, an inherently weak foot placed in an improper set of circumstances may be prone to develop underrun heels. In addition to genetics, the most common factor incriminated in the development of underrun heel syndrome is poor trimming, shoeing practices, and

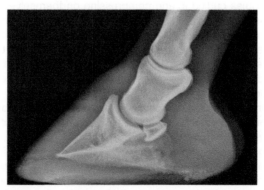

Fig. 4. Negative palmar angle of distal phalanx associated with underrun heels and dorsiflexion of the distal interphalangeal joint.

occupation,[2,19] although other factors may contribute. Inadequate removal of redundant toe, leaving the horse too long in the toes and setting the shoe too far dorsally, or shoeing short in the heels may initiate or perpetuate the development of underrun heels. Allowing too much time between shoeing can create the same scenario in horses prone to this syndrome. Failure to remove faulty horn at the heel that has undergone collapse or separation also perpetuates development of the condition. Two likely contributing factors not often mentioned are the level of work the horse is in and the environment in which the horse resides. Frequently underrun heels worsen in horses in heavy exercise, such as race training, without a change in shoeing practices.

The environment in which a horse resides may be important in the development of underrun heels. Horses that stand in moisture, such as urine and manure, generally have soft and weak horn. Daily bathing may also contribute. This weakened, soft horn combined with the stress placed on the foot during training may compound the collapse of the horn tubules.

EVALUATION

The clinical evaluation should begin with a detailed history of the patient, including the signalment, breed, age, occupation, and intensity and type of exercise. The duration and progression of the underrun heels and prior shoeing practices should be documented. The presence or absence of previous or current lameness, all prior diagnostic procedures, treatment, and response to therapy is also critical information. In addition, a history of accompanying problems, related to the hoof or musculoskeletal system or general health status, is essential and may influence case management.

After obtaining a detailed history, evaluation begins with a general visual inspection of the foot relative to the rest of the horse. Note the overall size, mass, angle, balance, and symmetry of the foot. Examine the positional axis of the foot under load relative to the bony column and the hoof-pastern axis in a neutral standing position and during locomotion. Determine the contact point of the heels relative to the hoof-pastern axis and the heel mass. Also observe the angle and relative strength of the fetlock and pastern by assessing the length and slope. After evaluation at rest, it is important to evaluate the length and slope of the pastern at varying speeds/gaits, because the contact point of the foot and the position of the hoof axis and contact symmetry are more accurately determined under full load bearing during locomotion than at rest. It is also vital to observe the way in which the foot travels and lands to accurately assess not only the severity of the condition but also the propensity for development of secondary problems, such as sheared heels.

After a thorough examination of the foot itself, observe the type of shoe applied, how it fits the foot, and the duration of time the shoe has been in place. It is important to inspect the shoe for uneven wear and the foot for overgrown areas of wall. Determine the angle of the hoof at the toe and at the heel while the shoe is in place. Measure both the length of the hoof at the toe and heel as well as the height of the hoof at the coronary band at both the toe and the heel to establish a baseline and assist in gauging therapy. A toe length to heel length ratio of greater than 3:1 has been proposed as consistent with an underrun heel[5] although this is not universally accepted as a definition. Note the location of the point of the heels of the shoe relative to the foot and their position relative to the widest point of the frog. Also observe the palmar point of the heels, which corresponds to the palmar process of the distal phalanx, relative to the heel bulb and to the position of the frog.

Examine the growth pattern of the wall and the level at which the curvature begins as well as the severity of the tubular curvature and degree of collapse. Inspect the bars and carefully pare this region to assess for bruising, scarring, or undermining of the sole or wall. Thorough evaluation with hoof testers and palpation of the hoof, coronary band, and digital cushion should be performed, noting any inflammatory signs, such as heat, increased digital pulse, and focal areas of pain. Visually note the general condition, thickness, and integrity of the hoof wall, especially through the heel and quarters.

The sole should be inspected for contour, degree of concavity, thickness, and integrity. Frequently the sole lacks normal concavity and becomes thinned and bruised. The contour and general health and position of the frog and digital cushion should also be evaluated. Often, atrophy and prolapse of this area occur with the progression of the syndrome.

Although the focus of the examination is the foot, it is also important to evaluate the horse in general. Make note of the environmental conditions in which the horse resides and record the body condition, any other conformational flaws, and any musculoskeletal disease that may be present. All of these parameters are considered when developing the most appropriate therapeutic management plan for the each patient.

After the physical examination, radiographic evaluation of the foot is a particularly useful adjunct and provides information pertinent to the development of an appropriate treatment plan for each individual.[17] The first radiographic feature relevant to underrun heels is the position of the distal phalanx inside the hoof capsule. Focus on the alignment of the bone relative to the dorsal wall and especially note the angle of the solar margin of the distal phalanx. Other important parameters include laminar thickness and sole depth. Changes, such as pedal osteitis, bony resorption, or proliferative changes, especially through the heel area, are also significant if present. Radiographs may also be used to determine the contact point of the heels relative to the hoof pastern axis and to confirm the hoof pastern axis determined in the clinical examination in a neutral standing position. Radiographs are also useful to determine intracapsular anatomic abnormalities not appreciated clinically.

If lameness is evident, it should be isolated as specifically as possible. The character of limb flight and the manner of foot contact with the ground aid in determining the source of the lameness and are crucial in prescribing treatment. Hoof-tester evaluation may clarify the region of the foot associated with unsoundness and is an integral part of the diagnostic process. Further isolation of the lameness may be performed with local anesthesia. Experience suggests a higher incidence of lameness associated with the medial heel than the lateral heel in the thoroughbred racehorse. Thus, peripheral distal limb anesthesia should begin with a medial uniaxial palmar digital nerve block unless the horse tests positive to the lateral heel. If lower limb anesthesia does not eliminate the lameness, it is possible that underrun heels are secondarily associated with the lameness. Whether a primary or secondary association is discovered, the distortion should be rectified.

Differentiating sources of pain directly associated with underrun heels may be difficult. The clinical evaluation should aid in isolating the source of pain and may be suggestive of the tissue involved but may not distinguish between soft tissue and bone. Ancillary diagnostic aids, such as nuclear scintigraphy, ultrasonography, or MRI, may be necessary to specifically identify pathology within the hoof capsule. Laminar disruption, sole bruising, digital cushion pathology, bone, and ligament or tendon involvement are possible.

TREATMENT/FARRIERY

There exits a great deal of controversy among farriers and veterinarians regarding proper treatment of underrun heels, which suggests there is no single best way to manage the condition. In large part, treatment options are provided by empiricism and reported testimonial data with little research documenting the efficacy of various proto-cols. The most successful treatments for underrun heels are associated with early inter-vention, before severe tubule deformation or hoof wall distortion. Due to the high incidence of underrun heels in racing thoroughbreds, however, lameness or severe distortion often predates recognition of the distortion as a problem. Most experienced clinicians agree that rapid resolution of the complex is not possible, and, therefore, the owner or trainer must make a long-term commitment when battling this syndrome. Chances for a positive outcome may be improved through vigilant hoof care. Individuals that have suffered a significant loss of tissue mass through the heels may never fully recover and are likely to become chronic management cases.

General treatment goals for managing underrun heels include maintaining sound-ness and function of the foot as well as establishing a normal hoof capsule with a normal angle, balance, and orientation. The theory for this correction is simple, and although correction in a static model is relatively easy, application under occupa-tion may be difficult. Realistically, the approach to therapy for underrun heels is largely determined by the severity of the distortion, the work schedule, and intended use, although other factors may play a role. Unfortunately, there are no biomechanical studies defining precise measurements that should be adhered to when addressing the feet; thus, experience is generally the guide when attempting to correct or modify the hoof capsule distortion.

Although the patient is in the midst of a rigorous athletic schedule, treatment gener-ally has 3 goals: to arrest the condition, to minimize the ongoing damage, and to prevent or eliminate lameness while maintaining the ability to perform. These goals are in contrast to a horse that can enter a long-term period of rest, where it is often possible to reverse the condition and restore a normal or near-normal hoof position, hoof angle, and tubular growth pattern. The contrast arises because it is possible only during a period of convalescence to take a global approach to management of the horse and control all factors involved in hoof growth, including biomechanics, amount of exercise, nutrition, and type of footing. This global control is not possible in horses that remain in work, although economic constraints of the owner, long-term goals for the horse, or the presence of other conditions may place lasting limita-tions on an athletic career and justify a period of convalescence. It is often possible to rehabilitate a foot to a healthier state during convalescence while barefoot, with appro-priate trimming and management practices. The period of time required to return the foot to a more normal state of balance is dependent on the degree of insult, the inten-sity of management, and the time of year.

Whether the treatment is palliative in the working horse or corrective in the conva-lescing horse, the goal is to use trimming alterations to facilitate regrowth and reorien-tation of the heels in a proper manner. Proper trimming is paramount to the recovery of the normal angles of the foot and is more important than the type of device applied to the foot. The hoof wall is trimmed with the goals of establishing a normal angle, balance, and length of the foot, and eliminating diseased or distorted horn.[13,17,20,21] A specific cookbook set of instructions is not applicable because there is notable vari-ation between feet; therefore, every foot should be treated individually. The first prin-ciple of appropriate trimming for underrun heels is to correct the overgrown toe. In general, this overgrowth in length is directed dorsally. Modification is achieved by shortening the toe and shifting the dorsal edge of the toe closer to the center of the foot (backing up or dubbing the toe) to establish a proper axis and position. This also facilitates breakover, which may be further enhanced by relocating the shoe pal-marly or rolling or rockering the toe of the shoe. Determination of the exact position of shoe placement for facilitation of breakover may be aided by monitoring the position of the distal phalanx radiographically.[4] It is necessary to establish breakover in a position that minimizes the forward pull on the dorsal lamellae to reduce the forward pull on the horn tubules of the heels. One should be cognizant that a significant amount of stratum medium is often removed, which has the potential to result in a loss of structural integrity and predispose to laminar bruising. Conversely, the removed horn is redundant and exacerbates the situation.

A second principle of appropriate trimming and management of underrun heels is to use healthy horn for heel support (**Fig. 5**). In order to achieve this goal, it is imperative to remove curved tubules and diseased horn; however, this may not be possible on an initial visit because if the condition is severe, this may create an excessively low angle, which has been shown associated with lameness. Several sessions may be required to achieve this goal and consistent re-evaluation is imperative to determine areas that may or may not be used during corrective trimming and shoeing. It is also critical to remain cognizant of the potential for overload of the remaining healthy horn. This risk is elevated if the horse remains at a high level of activity; care must be taken to avoid this circumstance because it perpetuates the condition and/or cause lameness.

A third principle integral to management of underrun heels is to dissipate load over a large area. This theory, combined with use of healthy horn for heel support, is the basis for many of the therapeutic shoeing techniques used in the treatment of this syndrome and is the basis for shoeing the foot as full as possible through the heels and extending the shoe caudally to the point where the heels ideally is located. Historically, egg bar shoes have been used for this purpose; however, the degree of extension creates a lever effect and concentrates the load on the edge of the heel, which exacerbates the problem (**Fig. 6**).[17] Straight bar shoes, heart bar shoes, onion shoes, roller motion shoes, heel plates, or other wide-webbed heel devices have been used successfully to support the heels during regrowth (**Fig. 7**). Implementation of these is often not practical for long-term use in a competing athlete. The addition of sole

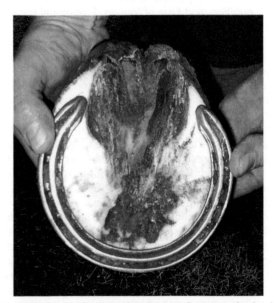

Fig. 5. Trimming to normal growth. Note the disparity between the heel of the previously worn shoe and the position of the shoe after appropriate trimming.

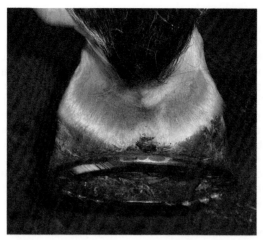

Fig. 6. Egg bar shoe. Note the potential lever effect due to the length of the shoe.

support in the form of pour-in pads (Vettec, Oxnard, California), or impression material, is often used to provide stability and protect the sole; however, this often results in overload and exacerbates the distortion of the heel.

Establishment of a normal hoof angle may require elevating the heels with a wedge pad, using a shoe with a built-in wedge, or using reconstruction of the heel with composite material. These practices have the potential for placing excessive load on the heels, and exacerbating the problem, however, may be necessary to combat secondary lameness problems associated with the low angle during convalescence.

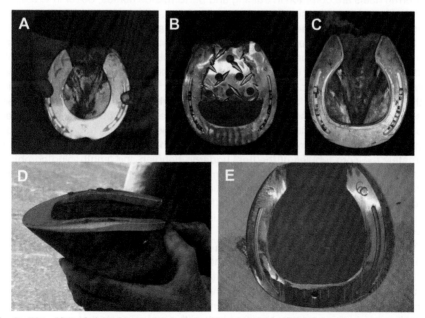

Fig. 7. Examples of therapeutic shoes: (*A*) wide-webbed aluminum support shoe, (*B*) heel and frog plate insert, (*C*) wide-webbed onion heel shoe, (*D*) roller motion shoe, and (*E*) wide-webbed shoe with pour-in pad. (*Courtesy of* Dr Bryan Fraley.)

Reconstruction of the heels with composite materials offers the advantage of recruiting other healthy wall for support and stability while achieving immediate restoration of form and function (Jerry Meling, Farrier, Lexington, KY, Personal communication, 2011). Theoretically, it is possible for new properly oriented horn tubules to grow while the horse remains in work, although this tenant is highly controversial and not universally accepted among farriers. A disadvantage of the technique is that there is potential for the horn degradation beneath the composite material, which can worsen the condition. This may occur in 1 or both of 2 ways: from overload or, theoretically, from moisture trapped in a confined, nonaerated space. Therefore, careful monitoring of the integrity of the heels is mandatory. Arguably this degradation is controlled through proper hoof preparation and application of the shoe. The horn must be clean and dry and the surface abraded by sanding. If this technique is used, the composite material must extend proximally to within approximately 1 cm of the coronary band and palmarly from the quarters to the point of natural heel contact to increase the surface area of attachment and maximize stability.

In conclusion, treatment of underrun heels is largely palliative, especially while a horse is in work. Long-term, conscientious hoof care is mandatory for re-establishing normal form and function of the foot to maintain long-term soundness. Corrective trimming is the primary focus of treatment and cannot be overemphasized, and shoeing practices are aimed at providing a protective role for the foot during regrowth. Considerations for exercise regimens and environmental controls, such as footing, housing environment, foot hygiene, and dietary management, likewise play a key role in long-term management of this condition.

SUMMARY

Underrun heels are common in training and performance horses, occur in virtually all working breeds, are unusual in pretraining juveniles, and may or may not be associated with lameness. Lameness is generally secondary in nature and may arise only as the underrun heels become severe or other distortion problems occur. Horses with underrun heels are predisposed to develop bruising, corns, abscessation, solar and wall separation, hoof cracks, sheared heels, subcapsular soft tissue injuries, and osteoarthritis of the distal interphalangeal joint and there is a possible correlation with navicular syndrome as well. In racing thoroughbreds, the condition has been associated with suspensory apparatus failure. The clinical presentation can vary broadly, depending on the severity of hoof distortion, presence of secondary problems, and degree of lameness. Etiology and pathogenesis are controversial but ultimately the horn tubules of the heel undergo bending and lengthening combined with loss of strength. The horn tubules may become parallel to the contact point of the ground and lose all ability to resist compression or absorb shock, accompanied by progressive dorsal shifting of the hoof axis. As the contact point of the foot moves further forward, tubular collapse is perpetuated and distortion of the hoof advances.

Patient evaluation, with special attention to all structures of the hoof capsule, is critical in developing a therapeutic plan for management of the syndrome. Radiographs are a valuable adjunct in assessing the distortion of the foot and response to therapy. Treatment may be palliative in the working horse or corrective in the convalescing horse, and goals include maintaining soundness and functional integrity of the foot as well as establishing a normal hoof capsule with a normal angle, balance, and orientation. Treatment of underrun heels should include trimming alterations to facilitate regrowth and reorientation of the heels in a proper manner. Proper trimming is paramount to the recovery of the normal angles of the foot and is more important than the type of device applied to the foot.

REFERENCES

1. Turner TA. Navicular disease management: shoeing principles. In: 32nd Annual Convention of the American Association of Equine Practitioners. Nashville (TN): American Association of Equine Practitioners; 1986. p. 625–33.
2. Chase BE. Underrun heels. Am Farriers J 1990;16(1):42–8.
3. Sigafoos R. Morphology, management, and composite reconstruction of the underrun heel. Am Farriers J 1990;16(5):26–37.
4. Dabareiner RM, Carter GK. Diagnosis, treatment, and farriery for horses with chronic heel pain. Vet Clin North Am Equine Pract 2003;19:417–41.
5. Turner TA. Shoeing strategies for palmar foot pain. In: 16th Congress of Italian Association of Equine Veterinarians. Carrara (Italy); 2010.
6. Moyer W, Schumacher J. Hoof balance and lameness: commentary. Equine Med Rev 1996;6:2.
7. Turner TA, Stork C. Hoof abnormalities and their relation to lameness. In: 34th Annual Convention of the American Association of Equine Practitioners. San Diego (CA): American Association of Equine Practitioners; 1988. p. 293–7.
8. Wright IM. A study of 118 cases of navicular disease: clinical features. Equine Vet J 1993;25:488–92.
9. Balch OK, Helman RG, Collier MA. Underrun Heels and Toe-Grab length as possible risk factors for catastrophic musculoskeletal injuries in Oklahoma racehorses. In: 47th Annual Convention of the American Association of Equine Practitioners. San Deigo (CA): American Association of Equine Practitioners; 2001. p. 334–8.
10. Kane AJ, Stover SM, Bock KB, et al. Hoof balance characteristics associated with catastrophic injury of Thoroughbred racehorses. In: 44th Annual Convention of American Association of Equine Practitioners. Baltimore (MD): American Association of Equine Practitioners; 1998. p. 281–3.
11. Eliashar E, McGuigan MP, Wilson AM. Relationship of foot conformation and force applied to the navicular bone of sound horses at the trot. Equine Vet J 2004;36(5):431–5.
12. Turner TA. Diagnosis and treatment of navicular disease in horses. Vet Clin North Am Equine Pract 1989;5:131–43.
13. O'Grady SE. Farriery for common hoof problems. In: Baxter G, editor. Adams & Stashak's Lameness in horses. 6th edition. Oxford (United Kingdom): Blackwell Publishing, Ltd; 2011. p. 1199–210.
14. Thomason JJ. Review of some past, present and possible future directions in biomechanics of the equine hoof. In: American Association of Equine Practitioners Focus Meeting on the Foot. Columbus (OH): American Association of Equine Practitioners; 2009. p. 41–65.
15. Decurnex V, Anderson GA, Davies HM. Influence of different exercise regimes on the proximal hoof circumference in young Thoroughbred horses. Equine Vet J 2009;41(3):233–6.
16. Peel JA, Peel MB, Davies HMS. The effect of gallop training on hoof angle in Thoroughbred racehorses. Equine Vet J Suppl 2006;36:431–4.
17. O'Grady SE. Strategies for shoeing the horse with palmar foot pain. In: 52nd Annual Convention of the American Association of Equine Practitioners. San Antonio (TX); 2006. p. 209–17.

18. Balch OK, Butler D, Collier MA. Balancing the normal foot: hoof preparation, shoe fit and shoe medication in the performance horse. Equine Vet Educ 1997;9: 143–54.
19. Moyer W. Therapeutic principles of diseases of the foot. In: 27th Annual Convention of the American Association of Equine Practitioners. New Orleans (LA): American Association of Equine Practitioners; 1981. p. 453–66.
20. O'Grady SE, Poupard DA. Physiological horseshoeing: an overview. Equine Vet Edn 2001;13:330–4.
21. O'Grady SE. Guidleine for triming the equine foot: a review. In: 55th Annual Convention of the American Association of Equine Practitioners. Las Vegas (NV); 2009. p. 218–25.

Farriery for the Hoof with a High Heel or Club Foot

Stephen E. O'Grady, DVM, MRCVS, APF[a],*,
Vernon C. Dryden, DVM, CJF[b]

KEYWORDS

- Horse • Flexural deformity • Club foot • Farriery
- Inferior check ligament desmotomy • Mismatched feet

KEY POINTS

- A club foot or flexural deformity may affect the horse at any stage of life from neonate through adulthood.
- The emphasis of this article is on defining and recommending the appropriate farriery for flexural deformities (club feet) which involve the deep digital flexor tendon and the distal interphalangeal joint.
- Clinical management of a flexural deformity is influenced by the severity, duration, and etiology of the club foot as well as the degree and source of lameness.
- There is limited information in the veterinary literature regarding the management of a mature horse with a club foot.
- The management of mismatched hoof angles remains a controversial subject for both the farrier and the veterinarian.

A horse with an upright foot with a high heel can fall within the realm of acceptable foot conformation, but this needs to be distinguished from a club foot. If measured, an upright foot will have a toe angle greater than 55°, the slope of the horn tubules in the hoof wall at the heels will approximate those in the toe, and the soft-tissue structures in the palmar foot will generally be well developed. The hoof-pastern axis will be parallel, the hoof-wall growth below the coronet from toe to heel will be even, and there will be no discernible distortion of the hoof capsule. This type of foot conformation can be bilateral or unilateral, whereby it is associated with so-called mismatched feet.

By contrast, a true club foot results from some degree of flexural deformity of the distal interphalangeal joint (DIPJ) that results from a shortening of the deep digital flexor musculotendinous unit.[1] A club foot or flexural deformity may affect the horse

The authors have no conflict of interest to declare.
[a] Northern Virginia Equine, PO Box 746, Marshall, VA 20116, USA; [b] Rood & Riddle Equine Hospital, Lexington, KY 40511, USA
* Corresponding author.
E-mail address: sogrady@look.net

Vet Clin Equine 28 (2012) 365–379
http://dx.doi.org/10.1016/j.cveq.2012.06.007
0749-0739/12/$ – see front matter © 2012 Elsevier Inc. All rights reserved.

at any stage of life from neonate through adulthood. A flexural deformity is character-ized by a shortening of the musculotendinous unit, which produces a structure of insufficient length to allow normal alignment of the distal phalanx (P3) relative to the middle phalanx, and results in variable mechanical changes within the hoof. These changes lead to the hoof-capsule distortions associated with a club foot. The farriery for a horse with an upright or steep toe angle is relatively straightforward and will be discussed briefly, but the emphasis of this article is on defining and recommending the appropriate farriery for flexural deformities involving the deep digital flexor tendon (DDFT) and the DIPJ. Flexural deformities of foals and mature horses are commonly referred to as club feet. Mismatched feet are also discussed at the end of the article.

ANATOMY REVIEW

In the antebrachium, the muscle bellies of the DDFT lie directly on the caudal aspect of the radius, and are covered by the muscle bellies of the superficial digital flexor tendon and the flexors of the carpus. The deep digital flexor muscle consists of 3 muscle bellies (the humeral head, the inconsistent radial head, and the ulna head), which form a common tendon proximal to the carpus. This tendon, along with the superficial digital flexor tendon, passes through the carpal canal and continues distally along the palmar aspect of the third metacarpal bone. Below the metacarpophalangeal joint, at the level of the middle phalanx, the DDFT passes between the bifurcating insertions of the tendon of the superficial digital flexor tendon, continues distally, and inserts on the flexor surface of the distal phalanx (P3). A strong tendinous band known as the acces-sory ligament of the DDFT (AL-DDFT) originates from the deep palmer carpal ligament and fuses with the DDFT at the middle of the metacarpus. The design and function of the anatomic structures is such that any prolonged shortening of the musculotendi-nous unit affects the position of the DIPJ. This palmar surface of the distal phalanx is pulled palmarly by this shortened musculotendinous unit, causing the DIPJ to flex. The alignment of the bone within the hoof capsule remains constant while the hoof capsule is pulled with the distal phalanx. The flexed position of the DIPJ combined with the altered load on the foot leads to a rapid distortion of the hoof capsule, and thus the club foot conformation. It can also be noted from the anatomy that transecting the AL-DDFT, when necessary, lengthens the musculotendinous unit either functionally or by allowing relaxation of the proximal muscle belly associated with the DDFT.

Classification of Flexural Deformities (Club Feet)

Flexural deformities have been classified as type 1 whereby the hoof-ground angle is 90° or less, and type 2 whereby the hoof-ground angle is greater than 90°.[2] A recent method of classifying flexural deformities using a grading system (grades 1–4) has been proposed.[3] It would seem beneficial to classify the severity of the flexural defor-mity so as to devise an appropriate treatment plan and monitor the response to a given therapy. A grading system would also enhance record keeping as well as improve communication between the veterinarian, farrier, and owner/trainer with regard to treat-ment strategies. A grade 1 club foot has a hoof angle 3° to 5° greater than the contra-lateral foot and a characteristic fullness present at the coronet. The hoof-pastern axis generally remains aligned. A grade 2 club foot has a hoof angle 5° to 8° greater than the contralateral foot, the angle of the hoof-pastern axis is steep and slightly broken forward, growth rings are wider at the heel than at the toe, and the heel may not touch the ground when excess hoof wall is trimmed from the heel. A grade 3 club foot has a broken-forward hoof-pastern axis, often a concavity in the dorsal aspect of the hoof wall, and the growth rings at the heels are twice as wide as those at the toe. A grade 4 club foot has a hoof angle of 80° or greater, a marked concavity in the dorsal aspect of the hoof wall, and a severe broken-forward hoof-pastern axis, and the coronary band from the toe to the heel has lost all slope and is horizontal with the ground. For simplicity, the first author uses a grading system based on the severity or degree of flexion noted in the DIPJ on the lateral radiographic projection to classify flexural deformities.

Flexural Deformities (Club Feet) in Young Horses

A brief review of flexural deformities in the young horse is presented here as an overview of this topic. Flexural deformities in foals can be divided into congenital or acquired deformities.[4–8] As such, congenital deformities are noted at birth, and acquired deformities generally occur during the first 6 to 8 months of life as the foal grows and develops. It is commonly a unilateral condition but may affect both limbs. The etiology of this deformity is unknown, but speculated causes include genetic predisposition, improper nutrition (ie, overfeeding, excessive carbohydrate [energy] intake, unbalanced minerals in the diet), and excessive exercise. A recent study looked at grazing patterns in a small number of foals, and showed that foals with long legs and short necks had a tendency to graze with the same limb protracted.[9] Fifty percent of the foals developed uneven feet with a higher heel on the protracted limb, leading researchers to believe there may be a possible correlation between conformational traits and an acquired flexural deformity. It is the first author's opinion that a major contributing factor to this syndrome is contraction of the muscular portion of the musculotendinous unit caused by a response to pain, the source of which could be physeal dysplasia or trauma from foals exercising on hard ground. Discomfort may follow aggressive hoof trimming whereby excessive sole is removed, rendering the immature structures within the hoof capsule void of protection and susceptible to trauma and bruising. Any discomfort or pain in the foot or lower portion of the limb coupled with reduced weight bearing on the affected limb appears to cause the flexor muscles to contract, leading to an altered angulation of the DIPJ. This shortening of the musculotendinous unit shifts weight bearing to the dorsal half of the foot, causing a decrease in sole depth and possible bruising of the sole, reduced horn growth of the dorsal aspect of the hoof wall, and excessive hoof wall growth at the heel to compensate for the shortening of the musculotendinous unit. The first clinical sign recognized is an upright appearance of the foot combined with the inability of the heels to contact the ground, especially after trimming the foot. As the condition progresses, the coronary band develops a square or full appearance dorsally. As the toe wears, the upright nature of the foot becomes more evident and the hoof wall assumes a straighter slope, losing its flare as it grows distally. The dorsal hoof wall begins to show a concavity and the sole-wall junction (white line) on the solar surface of the foot begins to widen. The toe of the hoof may become bruised and ultimately abscess, resulting in severe lameness. Differentiation should be made between a developing club foot and a foot where the dorsal hoof wall is upright from excessive wear at the toe. The upright foot is generally self-limiting as long as lameness is not severe or there is no abscessation. If lameness is present, a protective device (toe cap formed from a composite) over the toe will generally alleviate the problem once the foot grows sufficiently. A foot of this type responds well to appropriate farriery whereby the heels of the hoof capsule and the frog are trimmed such that they are kept on the same plane.

Clinical management of the flexural deformity is influenced by the severity, duration, and etiology of the club foot as well as the degree and source of lameness, if present. Evaluation of the foot should be performed at rest and in motion. The angle and the amount of hoof capsule distortion should be determined, and the foot should be inspected for under-run or separated wall or sole. Sensitivity to hoof testers or response to firm pressure from fingers over the dorsal sole should be assessed. If lameness is present, peripheral nerve blocks should be performed to isolate the origin of the lameness.

Radiographs should be used to confirm the diagnosis and assess changes in the joint. The first author administers mild sedation (half the recommended dose of xylazine [0.165–0.22 mg/kg intravenously] combined with butorphanol [0.011–0.033 mg/kg intravenously]) and places each of the foal's feet on separate wooden blocks of equal height, which allows normal loading of both forefeet. Lateral-to-medial and weight-bearing (horizontal) dorsopalmar views of both forefeet should be obtained. The degree of flexion of the DIPJ, the angle of the dorsal hoof wall, the position of the distal phalanx, and abnormalities at the margin of the distal phalanx should be noted.

TREATMENT
Mild Flexural Deformities

Conservative treatment, such as correcting the nutritional status of the foal (ie, weaning the foal to avoid possible excessive nutrition from the mare), restricting exercise to reduce trauma, judiciously administering a nonsteroidal anti-inflammatory agent to relieve pain, administering oxytetracycline to facilitate muscle relaxation, and carefully trimming the hoof is a good starting point. Hoof trimming begins with lowering the heels from the middle of the foot palmarly until the hoof wall at the heels and the frog are on the same plane. The bars should be thinned or removed, and the heels adjacent to the sulci should be angled to 45° to promote spreading. If sole depth is sufficient, breakover is moved palmarly. This action is accomplished by creating a mild bevel with a rasp that begins just dorsal to the apex of the frog and extends to the perimeter of the dorsal aspect of the hoof wall. If improvement is noted, this trimming regime is best performed at 2-week intervals. If the toe is constantly being bruised or undergoing abscessation, a hoof composite (Equilox or Vettec) can be applied to the dorsal aspect of the sole and the distal dorsal aspect of the hoof wall, to form a toe "cap" to provide protection.

Severe Flexural Deformities

A mild acquired flexural deformity may progress in severity despite conservative treatment, or a severe acquired flexural deformity may be acute in onset (**Fig. 1**). When a severe flexural deformity is present and confirmed during radiographic examination of the feet, conservative treatment and hoof trimming alone are generally of little benefit. Elevating the heels has been advocated, after trimming the foot, to reduce tension in the DDFT and to promote weight bearing on the entire solar surface of the hoof. Although elevating the heels improves the hoof-pastern axis and makes the foal more comfortable initially, the authors have not been able to subsequently lower the heel or to remove the wedge and establish a normal hoof angle with the heel on the ground. Once a marked flexural deformity of the DIPJ and distortion of the hoof capsule is present or occurring, the authors recommend transection of the AL-DDFT combined with the appropriate farriery.[10,11] The second author's opinion is that the most positive results have been seen when this procedure is performed before the horse is 1 year old. The heels are lowered from the point of the frog palmarly, until the sole adjoining the hoof wall (sole plane) at the heels becomes solid. Any concavity in the dorsal aspect of the hoof wall is removed with a rasp. Rather than a toe extension, a composite mixed with fiberglass strands is applied to the solar

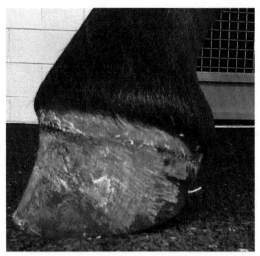

Fig. 1. Grade 3 club foot showing a marked flexural deformity with the heel off the ground. (*Courtesy of* Vernon C. Dryden, DVM, CJF, Lexington, KY.)

surface of the foot, beginning at the apex of the frog and extending to the perimeter of the hoof wall, where a thin lip is formed. The composite is molded into a wedge starting at 0° at the apex of the frog and extending to 2° to 3° at the toe (**Fig. 2**).[12] The wedge affords protection for the toe region, appears to redistribute the load to the palmar aspect of the foot, increases the stresses on the DDFT, and restores the concavity to the sole. This composite is not an extension, and only aids in protecting the compromised solar region of the toe while the hoof rehabilitates. It is advantageous not to

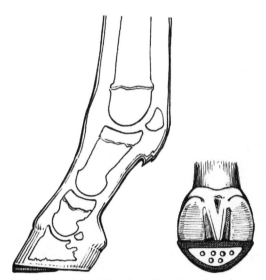

Fig. 2. Illustration of the lateral side of the foot after trimming, showing the placement of a reverse wedge. Illustration of the ground surface of the foot shows the composite wedge reinforced with an aluminum plate. (*Courtesy of* Stephen E. O'Grady, DVM, MRCVS, APF, Marshall, VA.)

apply a toe extension but rather to help realign the distal phalanx with the middle and proximal phalanges.

Flexural Deformities in the Mature Horse

Club foot

There is very limited information in the veterinary literature regarding the management of a mature horse with a club foot. An upright conformation of the foot associated with a flexural deformity of the DIPJ is defined as a club foot (**Fig. 3**).[1,4,13] A flexural deformity is generally diagnosed and treated while the horse is immature, but often a mild flexural deformity is ignored or the foal is treated inappropriately. When the horse enters training, the existing flexural deformity may become exacerbated by the type and amount of exercise, inadequate farrier care, such as inappropriate or infrequent trimming and shoeing, or some type of underlying disease. When a club-foot conformation is acquired in the adult horse, it is almost always secondary to an underlying cause or disease, such as an injury that results in a severe lameness; excessive trimming of the toe resulting in solar pain; chronic, low-grade laminitis; or chronic heel pain. Furthermore, flexural deformities have been reported as a cause of decreased athletic performance and chronic, low-grade lameness in the mature horse.[14,15] The altered biomechanics of the foot result in an increased load (ie, weight bearing) being placed on the dorsal section of the foot, leading to decreased sole growth, sole bruising, a shortened stride on the affected limb, and various degrees of lameness and poor performance. However, the majority of horses with a club foot maintain soundness, yet the club-foot conformation and the altered load on the foot may be responsible for poor performance.

Hoof-capsule distortion

To apply the appropriate farriery, understanding the proposed mechanism leading to the club-foot conformation is helpful. When a flexural deformity of the DIPJ is present, the musculotendinous unit is shortened, the degree of which is determined by the amount of flexion in the DIPJ. This shortening causes a disparity of hoof-wall growth, because decreased weight bearing by the heels encourages more growth at the heel than at the toe to compensate. The frog generally recedes because of the excessive

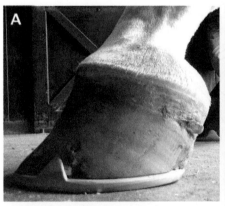 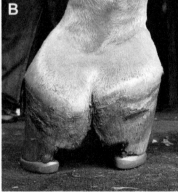

Fig. 3. (A) Lateral view of a grade 3 club foot. Note the broken-forward hoof-pastern axis and concavity in the dorsal hoof wall. (B) Palmar view of the same foot. Note the sheared heel on the medial side, the contracted heels, and the frog recessed between the hoof walls at the heels.

hoof wall growth at the heels, so that the energy of impact is assumed entirely by the hoof wall, bypassing the soft-tissue structures in the palmar section of the foot and transferring the load directly onto the bones of the digit through the laminar interface. The flexural deformity, combined with the excess hoof-wall growth at the heels, places the DIPJ in flexion and distal phalanx in an abnormal alignment relative to the digit, promoting toe-first landing, and excessive load is assumed by the dorsal section of the joint and the dorsal section of the foot. Hoof abnormalities associated with club-foot conformation are thin flat soles, poor hoof-wall consistency especially at the toe, toe cracks, hoof-wall separation, white-line disease, and chronic laminitis (**Fig. 4**).[16] Injuries associated with a high hoof angle are thought to include inflammation of the DIPJ caused by abnormal loading of the joint, sole bruising, and increased strain on the suspensory ligaments of the navicular bone.[17]

Radiology

Good-quality radiographs, consisting of a lateral-to-medial and weight-bearing (horizontal) dorsopalmar views, are necessary for the clinician and farrier to evaluate and treat a horse with a club foot. Good soft-tissue detail allows distortion of the hoof capsule to be accessed. A lateral-to-medial radiographic examination reveals the weight-bearing properties of the foot, the position of the distal phalanx within the hoof capsule, solar depth, length of the heels, the osseous integrity of the perimeter of the distal phalanx, and the severity of the flexural deformity of the DIPJ (**Fig. 5**). The degree of flexion indicates the amount of shortening of the musculotendinous unit. The radiographs are used to diagnose any abnormality present and to determine treatment options, and should be used as a template for farriery.

Therapeutic Farriery

Therapeutic farriery forms the mainstay of treatment for club feet. Farriery should be based on principles rather than a particular method, and the principles remain the same regardless of the severity of the flexural deformity.[16,18] The principles are to achieve normal alignment between the proximal, middle, and distal phalanges and, thus, normal orientation and loading of the distal phalanx relative to the ground. Trimming and shoeing is directed toward reducing weight bearing by the toe and dorsal aspect of the distal phalanx, and reestablishing weight bearing on the entire solar surface of the distal phalanx and the corresponding hoof wall. Historically, farriers have been taught to trim (lower) the heels to correct the distorted hoof capsule and promote weight bearing in the heel area, but this type of trimming comes with a price.

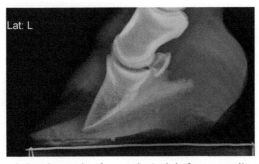

Fig. 4. Lateral-to-medial radiograph of a grade 3 club foot complicated with white-line disease and clinical chronic laminitis.

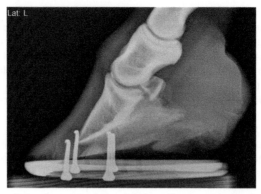

Fig. 5. Lateral-to-medial radiograph of the club foot illustrated in **Fig. 3**. Mechanically, note the load being placed on the dorsal section of the foot and the lucency just above the shoe in the palmar section of the foot corresponding to the recessed frog.

As the severity of the flexural deformity increases, it is proportional to the amount of shortening of the musculotendinous unit; therefore, lowering the heels directly increases the tension within the musculotendinous unit. These stresses may lead to further distortion of the hoof capsule, loss of sole depth, pedal osteitis, irresolvable tearing of the dorsal lamellae, and widening of the sole-wall junction similar to that seen in the chronic laminitic hoof.[19] The abnormal loading of the hoof often results in lameness.

Farriery

Distinguishing between an upright foot with steep hoof angle and a club foot is important. High hoof angles without phalangeal misalignment can generally be managed by adhering to good farriery guidelines for trimming such as using the hoof-pastern axis, the center of rotation, and trimming the heels to include the frog. It may be necessary with a steep toe angle to mildly trim the foot in a tapered fashion from the apex of the frog to the heels. This action increases the ground surface of the foot and attempts to reestablish weight bearing on the entire solar surface of the foot. Breakover is moved palmarly at the same time to compensate for any increased tension in the DDFT created by lowering the heels, which can be accomplished by rolling, rockering, or grinding breakover into the toe of the shoe. (**Fig. 6**) Horses with club feet should be trimmed/shod on a routine 4-week schedule.

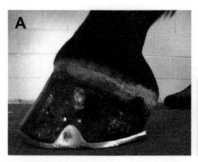
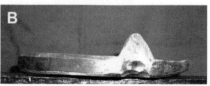

Fig. 6. (*A*) Grade 2 club foot with a rocker toe steel shoe. (*B*) Aluminum shoe with a forged rocker toe and slight wedge.

Farriery to correct a high hoof angle accompanied by a flexural deformity becomes more of a challenge. Again, the object of farriery is to load the heels, compensate for the shortening of the DDFT, and improve the hoof-pastern axis. To accomplish these objectives, farriery is directed at lowering the heels, but the amount to be removed can be difficult to determine. In mild to moderate club feet, an estimate of how much heel to remove can be made by placing the thick end of a 2- or 3-degree pad under the toe of the foot and allowing the horse to stand on it (**Fig. 7**). If the horse does not resent the tension it places on the DDFT, this test allows the farrier to safely trim the hoof wall at the heels in a tapered fashion starting at the toe or the widest part of the foot, using the thickness of the degree pad as a guide. The toe is shortened by trimming the outer surface of the dorsal hoof wall with a rasp. The trimmed foot is fitted with a shoe that has the breakover forged or ground into it, starting just dorsal to the apex of the frog and tapering toward the toe to further decrease the stresses on the DDFT. There are also commercial shoes with a rockered toe available that provide appropriate breakover. In cases with moderate to severe hoof-capsule distortion, lateral-to-medial radiographs are absolutely necessary to determine sole depth and how much toe can be removed to accommodate a rocker in the shoe.

With the more advanced cases of club feet, the heels should still be lowered to load the heels and unload the toe, but the addition of heel elevation following the trim is necessary to compensate for the shortening of the musculotendinous unit. The concept of lowering the heels with the trim then wedging the palmar aspect of the hoof back up is often not understood. When the heels are trimmed back to the widest point of the frog, the load-bearing surface area of the foot increases, which is necessary for normal function of the hoof. However, the musculotendinous unit must be accommodated and maintained without excessive tension, which is accomplished by decreasing the breakover and by adding elevation to the palmar aspect of the hoof. The degree of wedge that is applied often mimics the amount of heel removed, but in many cases may be less attributable to mechanical contributions made by rockering or rolling the toe of the shoe. The amount of heel elevation needed can be demonstrated following the trim by placing the trimmed foot on the ground 6 to 8 inches (15–20 cm) palmar to the contralateral limb (**Fig. 8**). A space will generally appear between the heels of the foot and the ground. A wedge shoe or a degree pad or a bar wedge is placed between the heels of the foot and the shoe to

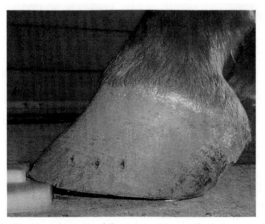

Fig. 7. Wedge pad placed under toe of foot to estimate the amount of heel that can be removed without excess stress on deep digital flexor tendon.

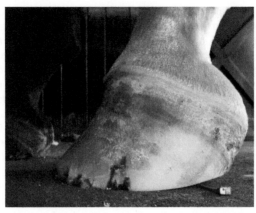

Fig. 8. Following the trim, the foot is placed palmar to contralateral limb to estimate shortening of the muscle tendon unit. Note the space between the heels and the ground.

compensate for the shortening of the musculotendinous unit (**Fig. 9**). This method allows the heels to be weight bearing but at the same time decreases the stresses on the musculotendinous unit. Creating breakover in the shoe to further relieve stress in the DDFT, as described above, is essential.

When the heels are elevated with a shoe, the normal ground-reaction forces and load-bearing structures are altered. To redistribute the load, it has been beneficial to apply a "pour-in" pad or impression material to the sole of the hoof to reestablish load sharing of the weight-bearing structures of the hoof. Without increasing the surface area over which the ground-reaction force is distributed, the heels may become overloaded over time and possibly result in quarter cracks, contracted heels, and subsolar bruising of the heel region.

Providing adequate heel expansion in the shoe may be beneficial as it may allow the club foot to expand, because most club feet have contracted heels (**Fig. 10**), However, keeping a shoe that is fit full in the heels on a club foot can be a difficult task because of the increased risk of the horse pulling it. In addition, a flat shoe with a roll in the toe can

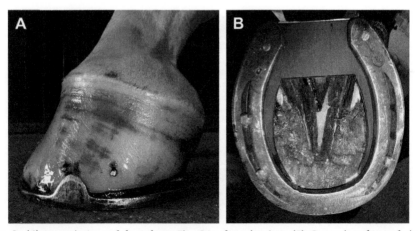

Fig. 9. (*A*) Lateral view of foot from **Fig. 3**A after shoeing. (*B*) Ground surface of shoe showing wedge insert and breakover created from the second nail hole dorsally.

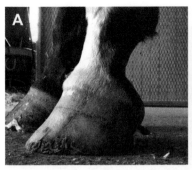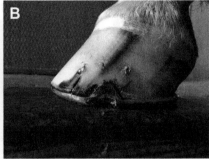

Fig. 10. (*A*) Grade 2 club foot pretrim. (*B*) After shoeing, with a rocker toe steel shoe.

be used after surgery and trim to provide protection and help maintain alignment while the hoof rehabilitates. Hoof-wall consistency may be so poor that alternative methods of application (other than nailing) must be integrated. Although different methods of shoe application are not covered in depth here, it is important to understand the methods available. The most common method of "glueing" a shoe on is called direct glueing. This method fixes a shoe directly to the weight-bearing surface of the hoof wall and sole via some type of adhesive. Aluminum rather than steel shoes are typically used for this purpose, because aluminum is very porous and the adhesives adhere with more affinity. The same principles for shoe fit are used with glue-on shoes versus shoes that are nailed. A drawback to direct glue-on aluminum shoes is that the normal expansion of the heels may be lost. Recently, polyurethane shoes have reached the marketplace, and can be applied via the direct glueing technique. These shoes are mentioned because they allow the heels to expand yet still carry the advantage of being attached with an adhesive. (**Fig. 11**). Although glue-on shoes will never take the place of traditional farriery, this alternative is often necessary to prevent the compromised club foot from continuing to lose sole depth and develop further hoof-capsule distortion by not having a shoe applied. It is always the goal, however, to graduate the horse into the most normal and simple shoeing/trimming protocol when possible.

Farriery Combined with Surgery

In selected cases, horses with a severe flexural deformity or horses that have not responded to appropriate farriery and remain lame may benefit from a distal check ligament desmotomy.[1,4,14,19] As a guideline for the practitioner, using the grading scale of 1 to 4, horses with club feet grade 3+ and 4 typically require an inferior check ligament desmotomy. This release procedure, along with therapeutic farriery, allows realignment of the distal phalanx within the remainder of the digit and readily allows the accompanying distortion of the hoof capsule to be improved. If this surgery is being contemplated, it should be performed early in the horse's athletic career, before there is a significant hoof-capsule distortion and before radiographic changes involving the DIPJ and/or the margin of the distal phalanx become evident. Again, it is of upmost importance to have good-quality radiographs of the digit before performing this procedure. It is also recommended to take follow-up radiographs after surgery and after trimming/shoeing to evaluate the digital alignment of the affected limb.

In the mature horse, the surgery can be performed under general anesthesia or with standing sedation/local or regional analgesia.[20,21] In the standing horse, the heel should be elevated by taping a 12-degree wedge to the foot to decrease tension in the inferior check ligament/DDFT complex allowing the check ligament to be easily identified,

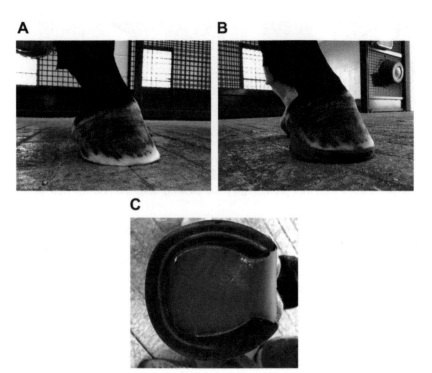

Fig. 11. (*A*) Adult grade 2 club foot. (*B*) Wedged rocker toe Polyflex shoe glued directly with Equilox. (*C*) Pour-in pad with Equi-Pak CS.

separated, and transected away from the cutaneous incision. The client should be forewarned that the surgery involves an extended recovery period, and a blemish or fibrous thickening at the surgery site is inevitable because of the mature nature of the tissue. Caution is advised when performing the farriery that accompanies the surgery, because the soft-tissue structures within the hoof capsule and the digit will have adapted/accommodated for the distortion of the hoof capsule. The authors trim the hoof in moderation and according to information obtained from the radiographs, and then apply 2 or 3 2-degree wedge pads using either a shoe or a cuff. After surgery the horse is walked daily, and a degree pad is removed every 7 to 10 days depending on the comfort of the horse. After 3 weeks the horse is allowed turn out in a small paddock for an additional 3 weeks and then is turned out in a larger area for 3 to 6 months before exercise is resumed. The cosmetic appearance of the limb is maximized by keeping the limb bandaged for the first 6 weeks. In a limited number of cases that the first author has managed or consulted on, the benefit to the horse in terms of a better prognosis for soundness far outweighs the labor-intensive nature of the rehabilitation process (Stephen E. O'Grady, unpublished data, 2011). The author has not realized any benefit in applying a toe extension to the shoe in the adult horse following surgery. Many mature horses with a club foot frequently have damage to the dorsal lamina similar to that found in horses with laminitis, therefore toe extensions may markedly exacerbate detrimental mechanical forces on the lamellae.

MISMATCHED FEET

The management of mismatched hoof angles remains a controversial subject for both the farrier and veterinarian. Commonly horses will present with feet that have a high or upright angle on one foot and a low hoof-capsule angle on the other foot (**Fig. 12**). Limb-length disparity has been suggested as a cause for mismatched feet, although it has not been scientifically proven. One study has suggested that 28% of normal performance horses have been affected by mismatched feet. The difference between the forefeet could range anywhere from a disparity between the angles of the dorsal hoof wall to a club foot on one limb and an overloaded low heel on the contralateral limb. Horses with a disparity between dorsal hoof-wall angles will generally have a straight hoof-pastern axis, and the hoof-wall growth below the coronet from the toe to the heel will be even. In this case, the authors suggest using good farriery principles to trim and shoe each foot on an individual basis.

Managing horses with mismatched feet whereby one foot has a markedly high hoof angle or a club foot becomes more complex. This type of case will often present with a shortened stride on the limb with the upright foot or a discernible lameness. The lameness may be observed in the contralateral foot from overloading the heel on that side, owing to the shortened stride placing excess weight on that foot over time. Overloading one limb verses the other can be seen in cases of chronic unilateral lameness such as a shoulder osteochondritis dissecans. The limb with the shoulder lesion will often develop a club foot caused by lack of weight bearing and shortening of the musculotendinous unit; this would be considered an acquired club foot. Conversely, the contralateral limb may overload and result in a flat "panned-out" low-angle foot. Managing these horses can be difficult, and the proper shoeing protocol may not be inherently obvious. If lameness is involved, diagnosing and addressing the lameness is the first step in the process. A common mistake made in this situation is to wedge up the low-angle foot to make it match the upright foot. The clinician may feel it necessary to add a wedge to the foot with a low angle simply because a wedge was added to the upright or club foot. The authors again recommend treating each foot individually, and to trim and shoe the foot using appropriate guidelines. The management of the club foot has been discussed in the previous section. When approaching the foot with the low angle, the clinician is often inclined to wedge up the heels to improve the hoof-pastern axis. However, this will place more stress on the already compromised heel structures. Although the hoof-pastern axis will appear improved immediately following the shoeing, the long-term effect is exacerbation of the low angle, further crushing of the heels, and prolapse of the frog below the ground surface of the foot. Alternatively, the heels should be trimmed back to the widest point of the frog if possible, or an attempt should be made to get the hoof wall at the heels and the frog on the same plane. As much toe length as possible should be removed. It is extremely important to obtain good-quality radiographs

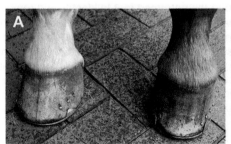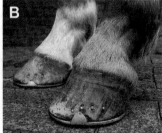

Fig. 12. (*A*) Dorsal view of a pair of mismatched feet. (*B*) Lateral view of same feet. Note the even growth rings and the straight hoof-pastern axis on the left forefoot. (*Courtesy of* Dr Marianne Sloet, Veterinary College of Utrecht, The Netherlands.)

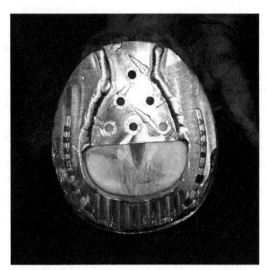

Fig. 13. Aluminum shoe with a heel plate and impression material used to help with load sharing of the weight-bearing structures.

before trimming to determine the amount of heel and especially sole that can be removed. If there is adequate sole depth available to allow a rocker toe to be trimmed into the foot, this is very beneficial to the biomechanics of the low-angle hoof. The center of force on a low-angle foot is further palmar than that of the upright or normal hoof. Therefore, the shoeing protocol is directed at moving the center of force away from the overloaded heels. In addition, load sharing of the weight-bearing structures of the low-angle foot may help to decrease the forces directed to the heels. This action can be accomplished with impression material, a pour-in pad, a plastic frog-support pad, or a heel plate added to the palmar aspect of the shoe (**Fig. 13**).

SUMMARY

The club foot is an important cause of equine lameness and a is challenge to the veterinarian and farrier. The clinician must recognize and understand the altered mechanics that are placed on the osseous structures within the hoof and on the hoof capsule that accompany a flexural deformity involving the DIPJ. This understanding allows the clinician to apply the appropriate treatment and appreciate subsequent improvement. In addition, it is essential to look beyond the deformed foot to identify and remove, if possible, any underlying cause. As with most disorders, early recognition and intervention significantly increase the chance of a successful outcome, which is especially true when dealing with the young horse. Knowledge, skill, and interaction between the veterinarian and farrier are necessary for a successful outcome when treating a horse with a flexural deformity, regardless of whether treatment is limited to farriery or is combined with surgery.

REFERENCES

1. O'Grady SE. Farriery for common hoof problems. In: Baxter GM, editor. Adams and Stashak's lameness in horses. 6th edition. Ames (IA): Wiley-Blackwell; 2011. p. 1199–210.

2. Adams SB. Management of congenital and acquired limb deformities. Proc Am Assoc Equine Pract 2000;46:117–25.
3. Redden RF. Hoof capsule distortion: understanding the mechanisms as a basis for rational management. Vet Clin North Am Equine Pract 2003;19:443–63.
4. O'Grady SE. Flexural deformities of the distal interphalangeal joint (clubfeet)—a review. Equine Vet Educ 2012;24(5):260–8.
5. Adkins A. Flexural limb deformity. In: Proceedings of the British Equine Veterinary Association Congress. Birmingham (UK). 2008;47:41–2.
6. Hunt RJ. Flexural limb deformities in foals. In: Ross MW, Dyson SJ, editors. Diagnosis and management of lameness in the horse. 2nd edition. St Louis (MO): Elsevier Saunders; 2011. p. 645–9.
7. Greet TR. Managing flexural and angular limb deformities: the Newmarket perspective. Proc Am Assoc Equine Pract 2000;46:130–6.
8. Kidd JA, Barr AR. Flexural deformities in foals. Equine Vet Educ 2002;14:311–21.
9. van Heel MC, Kroekenstoel AM, van Dierendonck MC, et al. Uneven feet in a foal may develop as a consequence of lateral grazing behavior induced by conformational traits. Equine Vet J 2006;38:646–51.
10. White NA. Ultrasound-guided transection of the accessory ligament of the deep digital flexor muscle (distal check ligament desmotomy) in horses. Vet Surg 1995; 24:373–8.
11. Caldwell FJ, Waguespack RW. Evaluation of a tenoscopic approach for desmotomy of the accessory ligament of the deep digital flexor tendon in horses. Vet Surg 2011;40:266–71.
12. Stone WC, Merritt K. A review of the etiology, treatment and a new approach to club feet. In: Proceedings of the American Association of Equine Practitioners Focus on the Equine Foot. Columbus (OH). 2009.
13. O'Grady SE. Basic farriery for the performance horse. Vet Clin North Am Equine Pract 2008;24(1):203–18.
14. Turner TA, Stork C. Hoof abnormalities and their relation to lameness, In: Proceedings of the 34th Annual Convention of the American Association of Equine Practitioners 1998. p. 293–7.
15. Balch O, White K, Butler D, et al. Hoof balance and lameness: foot bruising and limb contact. Compend Contin Educ Pract Vet 1995;17(12):1503–5.
16. O'Grady SE, Poupard DA. Proper physiologic horseshoeing. Vet Clin North Am 2003;19(2):333–51.
17. Turner TA. The use of hoof measurements for the objective assessment of hoof balance. Proceedings of the 38th Annual Convention of the American Association of Equine Practitioners 1992. p. 389–95.
18. O'Grady SE. Guidelines for trimming the equine foot: a review. In: Proceedings of the American Association of Equine Practitioners. vol. 55. 2009. p. 218–225.
19. Floyd AE. Deformities of the limb and their relevance to the limb. In: Floyd AE, Mansmann RA, editors. Equine podiatry. St Louis (MO): Saunders; 2007. p. 218–23.
20. Yiannikouris S, Schneider RK, Sampson SN, et al. Desmotomy of the accessory ligament of the deep digital flexor tendon in the forelimb of 24 horses 2 years and older. Vet Surg 2011;40:272–6.
21. Walmsley EA, Anderson GA, Adkins AR. Retrospective study of outcome following desmotomy of the accessory ligament of the deep digital flexor tendon for type 1 flexural deformity in Thoroughbreds. Aust Vet J 2011;89(9):265–8.

Farriery for the Hoof with a Sheared Heel

Stephen E. O'Grady, DVM, MRCVS, APF

KEYWORDS

- Horse • Sheared heels • Hoof capsule distortion • Limb conformation • Lameness
- Therapeutic farriery

KEY POINTS

- Sheared heels develop as an adaption-distortion of the hoof capsule as a result of an abnormal strike and loading pattern of the foot, which is generally a consequence of limb conformation.
- The growth rate around the circumference of the hoof should be approximately uniform, but regional disturbances in growth rate can occur to either increase or decrease growth.
- The primary conformational trait that is observed in horses that develop sheared heels is a rotational deformity of the distal limb and a narrow chest.
- Farriery is directed toward improving the hoof capsule distortion and decreasing the forces on the displaced side of the foot.

INTRODUCTION

A sheared heel is a very common and often overlooked hoof capsule distortion. The exact mechanism leading to this type of hoof capsule conformation is not completely understood and the farriery generally employed for sheared heels remains controversial.[1] Trimming and shoeing methods for sheared heels are often based on theoretical assumptions and opinions derived from empiric experience rather than an understanding of the basic mechanism that causes this type of distortion to occur. The shape of the distorted hoof capsule reflects the distribution of the load across the foot.[2] Sheared heels are also associated with an asymmetric strike pattern during the stance phase of the stride. It has become common practice to use the concept of dynamic balance when trimming sheared heels, which implies that horses should be trimmed such that the foot lands symmetrically or flat. The problem here is that the horse's leg conformation precludes achieving a flat landing pattern and trimming in an attempt to achieve it may be detrimental. This article will attempt to outline the etiology leading to a sheared heel conformation and present a rational approach to farriery.

The author has nothing to disclose.
Northern Virginia Equine, 8170 Patrickswell Lane, Marshall, VA 20116, USA
E-mail address: sogrady@look.net

Sheared heels as a clinical entity and a cause of lameness were first described in the veterinary literature 35 years ago.[3] A *sheared heel* is defined as a hoof capsule distortion resulting in a proximal displacement of one quarter/heel bulb relative to the contralateral side of the hoof.[4] The disparity between length of the lateral and medial quarters/heel bulbs is generally 0.5 cm or greater when the height of the quarters/heels is measured from the coronet to the ground or to the shoe. When the weight of the horse is not distributed uniformly over the entire hoof during the landing and/or stance phase of the stride, one section of the foot, usually a heel bulb and accompanying quarter, receives a disproportionate amount of the total load. The amount of displacement in the affected heel will be dependent on the amount of overload sustained by the individual foot. Sheared heels can occur in the hind feet as well as the forefeet.

THE CAUSE OF SHEARED HEELS

While the diagnosis of a sheared heel is straightforward, the etiology of the condition may be misleading and the farriery employed in the treatment is often based on opinions. Farriery or inappropriate farriery may play a role in the etiology because this hoof capsule distortion becomes more apparent in horses that are shod as opposed to horses that have not worn shoes. Limb conformation and the landing pattern of the horse appear to be the dominant factor causing this type of hoof capsule deformation. Sheared heels develop as an *adaption-distortion* of the hoof capsule as a result of an abnormal strike and loading pattern of the foot, which is a consequence of limb conformation. Trimming methods and the application of shoes may interfere with the adaption process and therefore potentiate the distortion. For example, with a horse with a shared heel on the medial side, trimming the quarter/heel lower on the opposite side of the foot, which is a common practice if the horse toes-out, will result in the hoof wall on the affected side being longer and accentuate the loading on that side. Prevention or possible treatment of abnormal limb conformation is only possible in the foal; therefore, in adults where conformation cannot be changed; therapy is directed toward managing the distortion of the hoof capsule.

SHEARED HEELS AS A CAUSE OF LAMENESS

The sheared heel receives a continuous repetitive disproportionate amount of the load, which results in the hoof capsule distortion. At the same time, there are increased stresses placed on the submural tissue in this area that predispose the foot to various injurious conditions such as:

- Unilateral palmar foot pain
- Hoof wall separations
- Subsolar bruising/corns
- Quarter and heel cracks
- Fracture of the bar
- A deep fissure within the base of the frog

In fact, seldom is one of the above conditions present on one side of the foot when not accompanied by a sheared, contracted, or under-run heel. It is also rare to find a quarter crack that does not have a sheared heel on the side of the foot with the defect. The pathologic developments that occur in association with this condition may be a major contributor to the palmar heel pain complex. The author has documented a sufficient number of obscure chronic lameness cases involving horses with sheared heels that could be termed unilateral (uniaxial) palmar foot pain. These are horses with a chronic lameness that is resolved by a unilateral palmar digital nerve block placed on the side of the foot with the sheared heel. This type of case generally responds to appropriate farriery where the conformation of the foot is improved and the load on the affected quarter/heel is decreased.

STRUCTURAL CHANGES TO THE FOOT

The equine hoof capsule is a viscoelastic structure that has the unique ability to deform when weight is accepted uniformly.[5] However, if an unequal load is continually placed on one quarter/heel, over time, structural changes will develop. The increased load on one side of the foot causes the coronary band at the heel and quarter to move proximally and the hoof wall to assume a steeper angle; that is, the wall becomes straighter followed by contracture of the heels. The narrow heel will decrease the ground surface of the foot, resulting in a lack of expansion on that side of the foot, making the solar surface in the palmar/plantar section of the foot asymmetric. The excessive stresses in the wall will also create distortions of the wall; the hoof wall begins to "roll under" on the affected side, which further decreases ground surface under that area of the foot. Generally, the side of the foot that first impacts the ground develops a flare, possibly due to bending of the horn tubules (**Fig. 1**). Additionally, those structures located between the wall and the middle phalanx are also under stress and variably displace. As the coronary band displaces proximally and the wall becomes steeper, the affected wall moves closer to the median plane of the limb, so that the pastern no longer joins the foot at the center of the coronary band (**Fig. 2**). A recent study of horses with spontaneous quarter cracks showed the free margin of the ungual cartilage above the coronet at the site of the crack to be less than 15 mm, as a result of the proximally displaced quarter/heel.[6] This will impede natural movement of the ungula cartilage and therefore is likely to interfere with the abaxial movement of the ungual cartilage when the foot is loaded. This potentially decreases the natural damping mechanisms of the hoof by limiting expansion, which would in turn increase the stresses in the wall and the tissues between the wall and the distal phalanx.

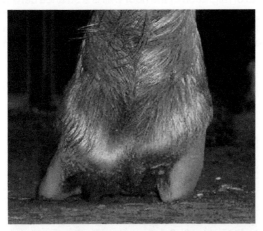

Fig. 1. Palmar view of a left forefoot with a medial sheared heel. Note disparity between medial and lateral heel length. Note the compression of the soft tissue structures proximal to the heel bulb, the flare on the lateral side and the medial heel starting to roll under.

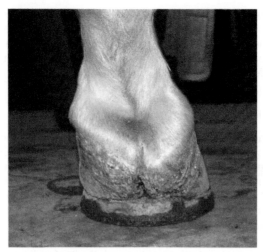

Fig. 2. Palmar view of a right forefoot with a medial sheared heel. Note the anatomic changes of the structures proximal to the heel bulb.

Secondary to the abnormal stresses and displacement of the coronary band, there is dorsal migration of the reflection of the hoof wall at its junction with the bar, which is readily apparent when the foot is viewed from the ground surface. Additionally, new growth of the hoof wall at the coronary band is suppressed, and therefore the growth rings below the coronet are tightly spaced. On gross dissection, the coronary groove, instead of being circular on a cross section, becomes distoproximally elongated and narrow in the displaced quarter/heel. The narrower coronet produces a thinner hoof wall in this area (**Fig. 3**).[1]

The growth rate around the circumference of the hoof is usually approximately uniform, but regional disturbances in growth rate can occur to either increase or decrease growth. The position of the coronary band is related to the balance between hoof wall growth at the coronary band and the rate of migration of the hoof wall distally. Furthermore, the rate of migration of the hoof wall is a balance between an active distal migration occurring within the lamellae and the force on the wall from the ground reaction force that tends to drive the wall proximally. Clinical evidence suggests that hoof wall growth is at least in part, if not predominantly, inversely determined by the force of

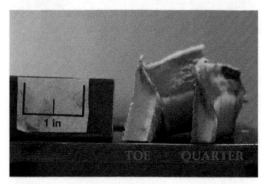

Fig. 3. Difference in the angle of the coronary groove between the toe and the quarter/heel on a horse with a sheared heel. (*Courtesy of* Mike Savaldi, Shandon, CA.)

weight bearing at the ground surface of the wall (Andrew Parks, personal communication, 2010); in other words, there appears to be a natural homeostatic mechanism whereby the growth at the coronary band equals wear at the ground surface and the force moving the wall distally is coordinated with that component of the ground reaction force that would move it proximally. If the force on the distal border of the wall exceeds the force that causes the wall to migrate distally or if the rate of hoof wall growth exceeds the rate of migration distally, the coronary band displaces proximally. This appears to be the mechanism in horses with sheared heels/quarters. The growth rings below the coronet are usually very close together where the hoof wall is displaced, which would be expected as a homeostatic mechanism to decrease hoof growth in response to increased weight bearing (force) by and proximal displacement/reduced distal movement of the wall. Whether this is a real phenomenon suggested by clinical experience has not been confirmed in a scientific manner.

THE ROLE OF TRIMMING AND SHOEING IN THE PATHOGENESIS OF SHEARED HEELS

For years it has been assumed that inappropriate farrier practices may lead to this type of hoof capsule distortion when trimming methods such as leaving the heels long or excessively lowering one side of the foot would result in excessive forces/stresses being placed on a given section of the foot. The term used to describe this type of hoof capsule distortion was a *lateral-medial imbalance,* and the proximally displaced coronet was often referred to by the farrier community as "jamming." The rationale for such a belief is at least in part that sheared heels are much more commonly observed on shod horses than in those horses that have been barefoot all their lives. Although trimming and shoeing may indeed contribute to a sheared heel, in the author's experience, it is not the predominant influence. It is reasonable to assume that trimming the heels unevenly during routine hoof care would lead to an abnormal mediolateral orientation of the hoof; however, both the viscoelastic nature of the hoof capsule and the pattern of hoof wall growth will compensate for this effect in a well-conformed limb.[5] To disprove the assumption that inappropriate poor trimming was the principal influence in the development of sheared heels, the author performed a small field study using a group of 25 horses (10 broodmares and 15 young race horses in training [most wearing front shoes]) on a large breeding farm to test this hypothesis. To enter the study, all horses had to have acceptable forelimb conformation such that using the carpus as a guide to assess the axial alignment of the limb distally; the limb was not rotated laterally. All the horses had to have a flat landing pattern on both forefeet when walked on a firm surface before their feet were trimmed. To test the hypothesis that trimming was not responsible for the development of sheared heels, one side of each forefoot was lowered (the medial side in most cases) relative to the contralateral quarter/heel every 3 weeks for 3 trims. Measurements of each hoof were taken at each ensuing trim and the position of the coronet was noted. In no instance during the study was a sheared heel able to be created or observed. Furthermore, with farriers having a thorough knowledge of hoof anatomy, the increased awareness of foot problems by the horse-owning public, and the continued improvement in the quality of farriery/farrier education, inappropriate trimming of the hoof does not appear to be the main cause or even a contributing cause of this condition today.

To further substantiate that trimming was not a primary cause of sheared heels, the author reviewed 50 dorsopalmar 0° radiographs on horses that had a foot with a sheared heel conformation where one heel bulb was displaced proximally 0.5 cm or greater.[7] In the majority of cases, it was clearly shown that the solar surface of the distal phalanx was approximately horizontal (parallel) with the ground. There was also an approximate amount of sole depth under both the lateral and medial palmar process of the distal phalanx. Furthermore, there was little or no disparity noted on either side of the joint space in the distal interphalangeal joint. The findings from this radiographic study would appear to be part of this remarkable process of adaptation. The study would further indicate the disparity in heel height was not originating from trimming practices applied to the hoof wall and sole located distal to the distal phalanx (**Fig. 4**). Anatomically, the distal phalanx occupies the dorsal two thirds of the hoof capsule while the majority of the space in the palmar/plantar foot is occupied by soft tissue (**Fig. 5**). The displacement of the coronet occurs palmar/plantar to the distal phalanx in the section of the hoof adjacent to the ungual cartilage. As the wall in the palmar third of the foot is supported by the ungual cartilage, the hoof wall displaces there in relation to the ungual cartilage just as it displaces relative to the distal phalanx dorsally. This also correlates with the decrease in the free margin of the ungual cartilage above the coronet that is observed with a sheared heel.

Conformation

Conformational faults in the upper limb that change the horse's flight phase of the stride appear to be the significant contributing factor leading to this type of hoof capsule distortion. Conformational traits that are observed in horses that develop sheared heels included rotation of the distal limb and a narrow chest. There is a far greater incidence of a sheared heel occurring on the medial side of the hoof but sheared heels on the lateral side are not uncommon. When viewed from the front, although the entire limb faces outward or, less frequently, inward, the axial alignment of the limb from above the carpus to the ground surface of the foot forms a straight line indicating a rotational deviation of the limb. An imaginary line drawn through the sagittal planes of each major joint will be aligned, indicating there is acceptable articular surface orientation through the joint. A lateral rotational deformity, where the knee faces laterally, will move the breakover in an outward or lateral direction, thus altering the flight phase of the stride such that the foot is unable to land evenly on both heels. Therefore, the altered flight pattern causes the horse to have impact with the ground

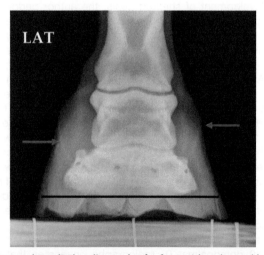

Fig. 4. 0 degree dorsopalmar (DP) radiograph of a foot with a sheared heel. Arrows placed at the coronary band of the heels show the different heel height, while the distal phalanx remains basically parallel with the ground. Note the distal phalanx in this radiograph is offset to the lateral side.

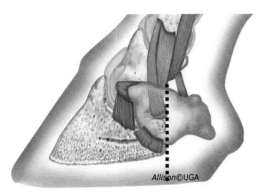

Fig. 5. Ratio of bone to soft tissue in the foot. The hoof capsule distortion noted in a sheared heel will involve the soft tissue structures palmar to the distal phalanx. Dotted line denotes the junction between the distal phalanx and the soft tissue structures of the foot. (*Courtesy of* Andrew Parks, VetMB, MS, MRCVS, University of Georgia, Athens, GA, USA.)

with the lateral side of the foot prior to full weight bearing. It is often hypothesized that this landing pattern predisposes the medial side to a greater load as the foot becomes flat; however, there is no research to substantiate this. More likely, this conformation predisposes the horse to greater loading on the medial side of the foot because the foot is offset in relation to the distal phalanx, but again there is no objective confirmation of this clinical observation. Using a slow motion video camera, one can actually distinguish the point where the foot impacts the ground on one side and the point where the hoof loads the surface on the other side.

It is a matter of interest that the lateral heel/quarter lands first yet the majority of sheared heels are on the medial side of the foot. When the foot is observed on the ground, the coronary band of the sheared heel appears higher, yet when the foot is picked up off the ground and the ground surface of the foot is observed in relation to the axis of the metacarpus, the lateral side appears longer. This can be attributed to conformation. It may also partly explain any role that trimming does have; namely, if the lateral wall appears longer with the hoof off the ground, it is more likely to be trimmed shorter, hence leaving the medial wall long, which is followed by the course of events described earlier. It will also cause the hoof to appear offset in relation to the pastern.

When viewed from the front, the hoof capsule often appears to be offset in relation to the pastern in horses with this conformation (**Fig. 6**). The presence of a sheared heel will make this appear even more so, so that the distance between the medial wall and the median plane of the limb is less that the comparable distance on the lateral side. On a radiograph, the phalanges appear to be aligned, but the offsetting of the hoof capsule can be observed with markers on the coronary band.

Observation

The evaluation of sheared heels begins with visual assessment of the hoof and limb conformation with the horse standing on a hard level surface. The gross changes noted in the foot are proportional to the amount of continual load sustained, the extent of structural damage, and the duration of the condition. When sheared heels are present, the heel bulb on the affected side is displaced proximally and the structures above the heel bulb will be compressed when viewed from behind the horse. When viewed from the front, the hoof wall on the affected side is straighter and, in chronic cases, will begin to roll under the foot. There is generally a marked flare of the hoof wall present on the side opposite the affected heel in the toe quarter, but a flare can often occur on the

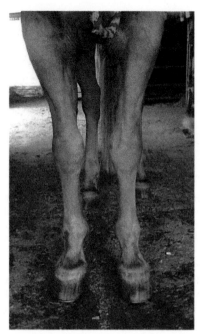

Fig. 6. Limb conformation associated with sheared heels illustrating a narrow chest, a severe lateral rotational deformity, and an offset foot.

side of the hoof with the sheared heel. When viewed from the affected side, the coronary band is displaced proximally above the affected heel and will assume a horizontal contour, or a focal displacement, instead of having a gradual uniform slope from the toe to the heel. The solar surface of the foot reflects changes elsewhere in the hoof capsule; the foot will be less symmetric; and the sole in the quarter and heel area will appear wider on the side with the flare and narrower on the side with the sheared heel.

It is important to view the horse in motion, again on a hard level surface from the front and rear. This should be done at a walk and a trot. When viewed from behind, this should determine which section of the foot is contacting the ground initially and which portion of the foot is receiving the excessive load as the distorted heel bulb will be obvious. When viewing foot flight and landing from the front, an airspace will be observed under the side of the foot with the sheared heel as it lands, again making the deformity more obvious. This landing pattern has caused much controversy as how the foot should be trimmed. The traditional concept that feet should be trimmed to land flat needs to be reconsidered as a lateral rotational deformity prevents the foot from landing flat. Attempts to make the foot land flat may result in uneven loading of the articular surfaces of the distal joints and will actually increase loading in the medial quarter/heel. The direction of breakover should be noted when viewed from the front. As the human eye is not capable of observing events of the duration of less than 20/1000th second, and foot landing and loading can be quite different at different speeds and gaits, slow motion review of high-speed film is highly recommended.

FARRIERY

Farriery is directed toward improving the hoof capsule distortion and decreasing the forces on the displaced side of the foot. This is accomplished by improving the shape of the hoof with the trim, improving the landing pattern and the application of the appropriate shoe. To improve foot conformation immediately, the author likes to remove the shoes, trim the heels lightly such that the hoof wall and the frog are on the same plane, and then stand the horse on a hard surface for 24 hours prior to trimming and shoeing the horse. This alone allows the affected side of the foot to settle into a more acceptable conformation. If a severe sheared heel is present, the unshod foot can be stood on some form of frog support and the foot is placed in a soak bandage for 24 hours.[7] Both methods result in a profound change in the hoof shape, and the distance between the coronet and the middle phalanx will widen. The author uses a double trimming method in an attempt to improve and unload the distorted quarter/heel. The foot is trimmed appropriately using the guidelines of a parallel hoof-pastern axis, the center of rotation and the heels of the hoof capsule trimmed to include the base of the frog.[8,9] To start the trim, a line can be drawn across the widest part of the foot with a felt tip pen. This is a good starting point as the center of rotation will be located just dorsal to the widest part of the foot. The frog is trimmed to where it is pliable and the quarters and heels of the hoof capsule from the middle of the foot are rasped palmarly so the heels of the hoof capsule and the palmar border of the trimmed frog are on the same plane if possible. An attempt is made to create as much ground surface under the affected heel as possible, which may result in the side with the sheared heel being marginally lower than the other side of the foot. This can be observed by sighting down the back of the foot; the hoof wall on the distorted side of the foot will be lower relative to the other heel and the base of the frog. The toe and quarters are reduced according to the sole depth so when the trim is completed, the surface area on either side of the line that was drawn or the widest part of the foot will approximate each other (**Fig. 7**). Lowering the heel on the displaced side of the foot is logical as it is the taller heel and it increases the ground surface of the foot on that side. Following the trim, the horse is again walked on a hard surface and

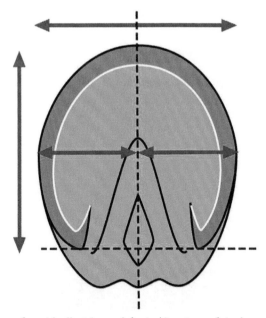

Fig. 7. Proportions of an ideally trimmed foot. (*Courtesy of* Andrew Parks, VetMB, MS, MRCVS, University of Georgia, Athens, GA, USA.)

some improvement in the landing pattern is generally noted. This may seem counter-intuitive to many, but it may suggest that part of the landing pattern is a compensation mechanism but the exact nature of this mechanism is unknown.

It is the author's opinion that when initially managing a sheared heel, especially when lameness has been localized to that section of the foot or if a quarter crack is present, the horse should be placed in a bar shoe if possible. Bar shoes effectively increase the surface area of the foot, allow the palmar/plantar section of the foot to be unloaded, and decrease the independent vertical movement at the bulbs of the heels. The author's choice is a wide web steel straight bar shoe (Kerckhaert Shoes, Shelbyville, KY, USA) fitted symmetrically to the trimmed foot (**Fig. 8**). Before applying the shoe, a second part of the trim is performed under the proximally displaced quarter/heel in a tapered fashion, which begins at the ipsilateral toe quarter (eg, inside toe for medial sheared heel) and extends to the affected heel. The amount of heel that can be taken off in the second trim depends on the sole depth at the seat of corn and on the severity of the proximal displacement of the coronary band at the sheared heel. The amount of heel, under the sheared heel, that can be taken off with this second trim ideally corresponds to the difference in length/height between the 2 heels. Lowering the hoof wall from the toe quarter to the heel will create a wedge-shaped space between the shoe and the hoof wall on the displaced side of the hoof (**Fig. 9**). This wedge-, or "pie-," shaped space created between the hoof wall and the shoe allows the distorted section of the hoof to descend to the shoe when weight is placed on the limb. This improves the landing pattern, unloads the affected heel, and allows the heel bulb to settle down and assume a more acceptable position. Feet with a low palmar/plantar angle rarely have enough sole depth under the affected heel for the second trim; in these cases, the rest of the hoof wall can be raised with a rim pad or with a full leather pad and impression material. When a full pad is used, impression material (Equilox Pink; Equilox International, Pine Island, MN, USA) is placed in the palmar section of the foot from the apex of the frog palmarly except under the displaced heel where the second trim was performed. Only the first 2 toe nails should be placed

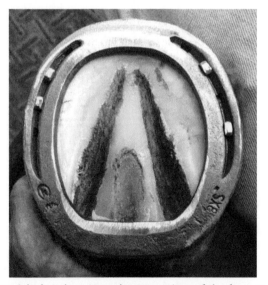

Fig. 8. Wide web straight bar shoe. Note the proportions of the foot on either side of the widest part of the foot and the breakover created in the shoe.

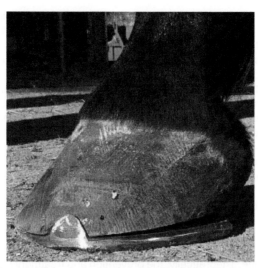

Fig. 9. Hoof wall lowered from toe quarter to heel on second trim. Note the tapered or "wedge-shaped" space created between the hoof wall and the shoe to unload the affected side of the foot. (*Courtesy of* Gabino Fernandez, Madrid, Spain.)

in the sheared heel side of the shoe to effectively allow the displaced heel to descend and settle into a more acceptable position. After the shoe is attached to the foot, the affected heel will rapidly descend onto the shoe when weight is placed on the limb, making the original space created by the second trim between the hoof wall and the shoe disappear. The extent of the second trim at the heel will determine the increase of free margin of the ungual cartilage above the coronet on the affected side of the hoof. This can be observed visually, palpated, and measured with calipers. As most horses with a sheared heel have a predisposing limb conformation (eg, a rotational deformity), these feet have a tendency to continue to deform the affected heel proximally and the double-trim method usually has to be applied to some degree at each consecutive shoeing. Horses with this type of hoof conformation should be reset at 4- to 6-week intervals.

Some cases will present with displaced heels that will resist lowering and widening of the sheared heel with the farriery methods described earlier. In these cases, a method is described that treats the distortion of the hoof capsule at the site of the sheared heel with a full wall thickness sub coronary groove, applied with a rasp or Dremel (Dremel Tool Co, Emerson Electric, Racine, WI, USA) tool about 20 mm below and parallel to the coronet.[1] Care must be taken to go all the way through the wall to the laminar corium, from the end of the heel forward to the most dorsal extent of the hoof distortion at the coronet. Horses may show mild discomfort from this procedure for a few days, especially if the laminar corium has been invaded, which results in tiny pinpoint hemorrhage being visible. Following the procedure, an antiseptic combined with a compressive bandage should be applied if necessary. The hoof wall growth proximal to the groove will show a totally new, wider, abaxial direction as it is disconnected from the stresses being placed on the straight distal wall.

DISCUSSION

Assessing the limb conformation, improving the foot shape, and applying the appropriate trim/shoe are essential when addressing sheared heel foot conformation. The heels of the horse's foot have a relative large amount of flexibility in the proximal to distal (vertical) axis. This can be explained by the *anatomic* features of the foot: a discontinuity of the hoof capsule between the heels with highly mobile structures interposed between, which include the frog, digital cushion, venous and arterial plexa, and fibrocartilaginous connective tissue. In other words, although the dorsal wall is intimately attached to the parietal surface of the distal phalanx, the laminar attachment or suspension in the palmar/plantar section of the foot is far less rigid. This provides the flexibility necessary for function but may also facilitate proximal displacement of the heels when these receive excessive stress or a disproportionate load. *Functionally,* this arrangement serves the bare-footed horse well as the hoof capsule at the heels is able to adapt to the uneven footing, but when shoes are applied, this ability to adapt becomes modified. When trimming or shoeing modifications in the saggital plane of the foot are being contemplated, it is important to be aware of this vertical mobility and the tendency for vertical displacement of the heels. A wedge pad under the heels, for example, will cause proximal displacement of the heels.

The prognosis for sheared heels is good, provided a skilled, interested farrier is involved. It is also necessary to have a committed owner as these cases often require ongoing maintenance. Theoretically, the prevention and treatment of lameness and/or quarter cracks, caused by a hoof capsule distortion such as sheared heels, are simple, but in practice they are often difficult to achieve. Being aware that there is a strong correlation between sheared heels and hoof wall problems, such as quarter cracks, makes prevention and treatment not only logical but imperative. When lameness is localized to a sheared heel or a hoof wall defect such as a quarter crack is associated with sheared heels, treatment becomes necessary, but sound horses with a sheared heel from any cause also will benefit from correction. Many times, improvement is all that can or will be achieved.

REFERENCES

1. O'Grady SE, Castelijns HH. Sheared heels and the correlation to spontaneous quarter cracks. Equine Vet Educ 2011;235:262–9.
2. Redden RF. Hoof capsule distortion: understanding the mechanisms as a basis for rational treatment. Vet Clin North Am Equine Pract 2003;19:458–61.
3. Moyer W, Anderson JP. Sheared heels: diagnosis and treatment. J Am Vet Med Assoc 1975;166:53.
4. Turner TA. The use of hoof measurements for the objective assessment of hoof balance. Proceedings of the 38th Annual Convention of the American Association of Equine Practitioners 1992. p. 389–95.
5. Parks AH. Form and function of the equine digit. Vet Clin North Am Equine Pract 2003;19:285–96.
6. Castelijns HH. Pathogenesis and treatment of spontaneous quarter cracks: quantifying vertical mobility of the hoof capsule at the heels. Pferdeheilkunde 2006;5: 569–76.
7. O'Grady SE. How to manage sheared heels. Proceedings of the 51st Annual Convention of the American Association of Equine Practitioners 2005. p. 451–6.
8. Snow VE, Birdsall DP. Specific parameters used to evaluate hoof balance and support. Proceedings of the 36th Annual Convention of the American Association of Equine Practitioners 1990. p. 299–311.
9. O'Grady SE. Guidelines for trimming the equine foot: a review. Proceedings of the 55st Annual Convention of the American Association of Equine Practitioners 2009. p. 218–25.

Farriery for Hoof Wall Defects
Quarter Cracks and Toe Cracks

R. Scott Pleasant, DVM, MS[a],*,
Stephen E. O'Grady, DVM, MRCVS, APF[b], Ian McKinlay[c]

KEYWORDS

- Equine • Farriery • Hoof wall defects • Quarter cracks • Toe cracks

KEY POINTS

- The mechanical behavior of the hoof capsule depends primarily on the physical properties of the materials that make it up and on its shape.
- It is well accepted that the hoof capsule adapts and changes shape according to how it is loaded.
- It is important for veterinarians and farriers to recognize the cause and effect of hoof capsule distortion.
- The management of full-thickness quarter cracks and toe cracks involves the identification and correction/management of balance issues and coronet displacement issues, unloading the injured region, stabilization of the hoof wall, and committed follow-up.

INTRODUCTION

The equine hoof capsule serves to support and protect the internal structures of the foot. Conditions that result in the loss of the structural integrity of the hoof capsule, such as full-thickness quarter cracks and toe cracks (full-thickness hoof wall fractures), are not uncommon and may result in lameness. Once the hoof wall has been fractured, the healing process is primarily replacement by growth. New growth originates from the coronet; depending on the region of the crack, it may take 4 to 12 months for the damaged hoof wall to be replaced. In most cases, healing by replacement occurs uneventfully if the underlying causes of the crack are addressed and the horse is allowed appropriate rest. The management of the underlying causes is paramount in reducing the likelihood of recurrence of performance-limiting cracks.

Disclosure: Ian McKinlay is principal owner and innovator for Tenderhoof Solutions LLC, PO Box 66, South Amboy, NJ 08879.
[a] Department of Large Animal Clinical Sciences, Virginia-Maryland Regional College of Veterinary Medicine, Virginia Tech, Phase 2, Duck Pond Drive (0442), Blacksburg, VA 24061, USA; [b] Northern Virginia Equine, PO Box 746 Marshall, VA 20116, USA; [c] PO Box 66, South Amboy, NJ 08879, USA
* Corresponding author.
E-mail address: rpleasan@vt.edu

Frequently, veterinarians and farriers encounter situations when it is important for horses with full-thickness quarter cracks or toe cracks to remain in work. These situations require the use of techniques that not only address the underlying causes but also stabilize the injured tissues. The purpose of this article is to discuss the predisposing factors for full-thickness quarter and toe cracks and to provide strategies for managing these hoof wall defects.

RELEVANT ANATOMY AND BIOMECHANICS

The equine hoof capsule comprises the hoof wall, sole, frog, and bulbs of the heel. The hoof capsule is made predominately of keratinized epidermal cells and forms a tough, obliquely oriented, truncated, incomplete cone that is folded in on itself on each side at the heels (**Fig. 1**A). The hoof wall is typically thickest in the toe region and becomes thinner and more elastic toward the heels. The medial hoof wall is usually straighter (less angled) and more upright (steeper) than the lateral hoof wall.[1]

The hoof wall comprises 3 morphologically distinct layers: the stratum externum (periople), stratum medium, and stratum internum (stratum lamellatum) (see **Fig. 1**B). The stratum medium makes up the bulk of the hoof wall and comprises the tubular and intertubular horn. The tubule density in the stratum medium is highest in the outermost region and declines toward the stratum internum.[2] This tubule density gradient reflects differences in the mechanical properties across the stratum medium and is

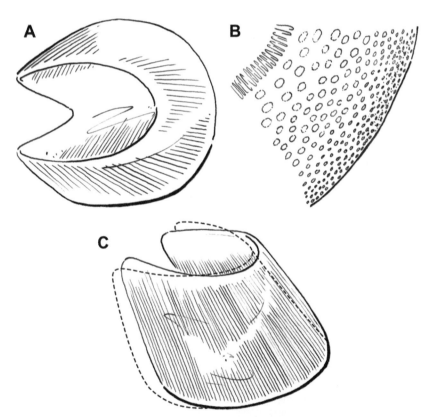

Fig. 1. The hoof wall: (*A*) shape, (*B*) layers, and (*C*) normal movement during loading.

proposed as a mechanism for modulating the transfer of energy from the rigid outer wall (high tubule density) through the more elastic inner wall (low tubule density) to the epidermal/dermal lamellae interface (and ultimately the distal phalanx). Also, the tubular-intertubular horn interfaces and the tubule zonation within the stratum medium have been suggested to be crack-stopping/diverting mechanisms, causing externally originating cracks to deviate along more tortuous routes and redirecting cracks away from the dermis.[3–5]

The mechanical behavior of the hoof capsule depends primarily on the physical properties of the materials that make it up (affected by nutrition and hydration) and on its shape (affected by load, limb conformation, and foot care).[6] During the stance phase of the stride, the hoof deforms under the weight of the horse and the dynamic loads of locomotion. The oblique, truncated, incomplete cone shape and the decrease in the wall thickness from the toe to heels in the well-shaped hoof causes the toe of the wall to bow backwards and the quarters and heels to flare at the ground surface (spread horizontally) during loading (see **Fig. 1**C). This pattern of deformation seems to be an extremely efficient mechanism for dampening and distributing the loads of weight bearing and locomotion. Changes in hoof capsule shape away from this ideal may negatively affect its mechanical behavior and predispose it to injury.[7]

PATHOPHYSIOLOGY OF QUARTER CRACKS AND TOE CRACKS

Many causes for full-thickness quarter cracks and toe cracks have been described, including coronet injuries, inappropriate farrier practices, poor-quality hoof walls (as a result of genetics, nutrition, or environment), white line disease, and hoof capsule distortion. In the authors' experience, the most common underlying cause of full-thickness quarter cracks and toe cracks is hoof capsule distortion. Accordingly, this discussion focuses on full-thickness quarter cracks and toe cracks caused by hoof capsule distortion.

It is well accepted that the hoof capsule adapts and changes shape according to how it is loaded. Hoof wall growth tends to be slower where most of the weight is borne and faster where the least amount of weight is borne.[8] Faulty limb conformation adversely effects how the hoof is loaded, and habitual disproportionate loading will change the shape of the hoof capsule over time. The resulting distortion of the hoof may negatively affect its mechanical behavior, resulting in abnormal stress and strain within its tissues. If the changes in stress and strain become excessive, the hoof wall will be predisposed to injuries, such as full-thickness quarter cracks and toe cracks. Stress and strain to the hoof wall may become excessive in a variety of clinical situations. Stress and strain may become excessive in horses with minor hoof capsule distortion but who experience high loads on their hooves (eg, heavy use or work on hard ground) or in horses with marked hoof capsule distortion but who experience normal loads on their hooves. In either situation, the underlying concept is that there is an imbalance between the load applied and the hoof wall's capacity to withstand that load. If the hoof wall stress/strain is excessive or repetitive, a full-thickness hoof wall crack may result.

It is important for veterinarians and farriers to recognize the cause and effect of hoof capsule distortion. This hoof capsule distortion may be multifactorial but the most common causes are poor limb/foot conformation and inappropriate farriery. Limb conformation directly affects hoof capsule loading, which affects hoof wall shape. For example, in horses with base-wide conformation (**Fig. 2**A), the medial heel quarter bears the most weight, which may cause the wall in this area to grow slower and become more vertical. If not managed properly, the medial heel quarter may

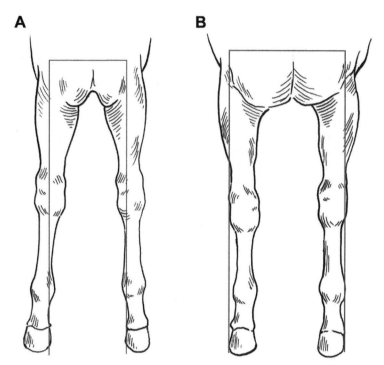

Fig. 2. (A) Base-wide conformation and (B) base-narrow conformation.

eventually become displaced axial to the coronet (roll under) and the coronet at the heel may displace proximally assuming a sheared-heel conformation (**Fig. 3**A). As a result of the disproportionate load, the lateral heel quarter seems to grow faster than the medial heel quarter, causing a distortion. The resulting hoof distortion negatively affects the mechanical behavior of the hoof wall, causing the medial heel quarter to bend axially at the ground surface and bow outward at the coronet during loading, predisposing to a full-thickness wall crack in the medial quarter region that originates at the coronet and extends distally some distance (a quarter crack) (**Fig. 4**). On close examination, quarter cracks usually open at the coronet when the foot is loaded and closes when the foot is unloaded. The resulting full-thickness wall crack usually results in performance-limiting lameness.

In horses with base-narrow conformation (see **Fig. 2**B), the opposite occurs. The lateral heel quarter bears the most weight, tends to grow slower, and becomes more

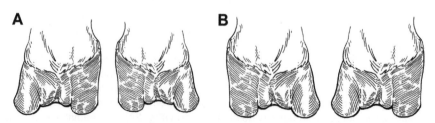

Fig. 3. (A) Hoof wall distortion associated with base wide conformation. (B) Hoof wall distortion associated with base narrow conformation.

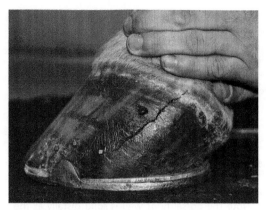

Fig. 4. Full-thickness quarter crack.

vertical. The lateral heel quarter may eventually roll under, and the coronet on the lateral side may displace proximally (see **Fig. 3**B). The resulting hoof wall distortion may result in abnormal bending of the lateral hoof wall that predisposes to lateral quarter crack formation.

Full-thickness toe cracks may occur in a variety of scenarios. The most common presentation is a full-thickness crack that originates at the coronet and extends distally. In these cases, the distal one-third of the hoof wall to the margin of the hoof capsule is usually solid. There is generally a proximal to distal concavity present in the dorsal hoof wall. The crack can be observed to open when the foot is unloaded and close when the load is applied to the foot. Full-thickness toe cracks are occasionally seen in horses with long-toe, low-heel conformation. This conformation loads the heels of the foot excessively, limiting growth at the heels and causing faster growth at the toe. This increased toe length creates excessive leverage on the hoof wall in the toe region during loading and especially at the breakover during the stance phase of the stride, predisposing to crack formation. Full-thickness toe cracks associated with this type of conformation usually begin as minor, incomplete cracks at the ground surface of the foot. If neglected, the cracks may propagate deeper and up the hoof wall and extend to the coronet. Lameness results if the crack fractures completely through the hoof wall, creating instability of the foot. It is not uncommon for toe cracks of this origin to be complicated by secondary white line disease.

Full-thickness toe cracks can also be seen in horses with excessively upright or clubfeet. In this scenario, the toe of the hoof may have a proximal to distal concavity and is loaded excessively. The coronet in the toe region may displace proximally as a result. Toe cracks as a result of this type of conformation/abnormal loading usually originate at or just below the coronet (in a manner similar to that of quarter cracks). The exact mechanism as to how a full-thickness toe crack occurs is unknown. As opposed to a quarter crack, a full-thickness toe crack will close when the load is placed on the hoof capsule and open when the weight is removed from the foot. There seems to be a reciprocal mechanism between expansion (or lack thereof) of the heels and movement of the defect at the coronet. At the origin of the toe crack, there will generally be a focal arch above the defect and one side of the crack may have an overriding appearance at the site of the defect (**Fig. 5**).

Full-thickness quarter and toe cracks occur almost exclusively in the front feet, presumably because front feet bear more weight than the hind feet.

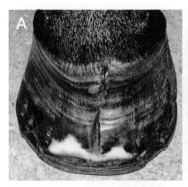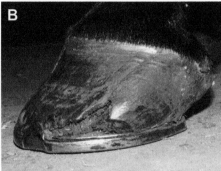

Fig. 5. (A) A full-thickness toe crack that shows focal displacement of the coronet at the origin of the defect. Note the dorsal hoof wall is solid distally at the ground surface. (B) Lateral view of same foot. Note the foot conformation, the concavity in the dorsal hoof wall, and the overriding margins of the crack.

MANAGEMENT OF QUARTER CRACKS

The management of full-thickness quarter cracks involves the identification and correction/management of balance issues and coronet displacement issues, unloading the injured region, stabilization of the hoof wall, and committed follow-up. In all cases, every effort should be made to identify the cause of the crack; if not, treatment success will be limited and the crack will likely reoccur. The assessment should begin with an evaluation of the horse's limb and hoof conformation, noting any cause and effect of limb conformation on hoof loading and hoof capsule conformation/distortion that would predispose to crack formation. Base-wide and base-narrow conformation should be evaluated and, if present, the effects on hoof capsule loading and shape noted. The presence of excessively vertical heel quarters, rolled under heel quarters, and displaced coronets on the overloaded side of the hoof should be determined. A focal prominence of coronet displacement is often present just above the origin of the crack, indicating the point of maximal abnormal stress/strain. Zero-degree horizontal dorsopalmar and lateromedial radiographs centered on the solar margin of the distal phalanx can be helpful in evaluating hoof capsule/distal phalanx alignment. In horses with quarter cracks, there may be inappropriate medial to lateral orientation of the distal phalanx relative to the ground. If medial to lateral imbalance of the distal phalanx is present, it may match the coronet displacement (ie, the distal phalanx tilts in the same plane as the cornet displacement) or be opposite of the coronet displacement (ie, the distal phalanx tilts in the opposite plane of the coronet displacement) (Fig. 6). When the distal phalanx imbalance is opposite of the coronary band displacement, it is likely the result of disproportionate loading on one side of the hoof causing faster hoof growth on the side of the foot where the least amount of weight is borne and slower growth on the side where the most weight is borne.

Affected feet should be trimmed appropriately using the guidelines of a parallel hoof-pastern axis, center of articulation bisecting the weight bearing surface of the foot, and the heels of the hoof capsule extending to the base of the frog or trimming the heel area to ensure the frog and the hoof wall are on the same plane.[9] If medial to lateral imbalance is present, the feet should also be trimmed in an attempt to realign the solar margin of the distal phalanx parallel to the ground. The amount of correction that is possible at any given trimming is dictated by the amount of sole depth available. It is acknowledged that complete correction of medial to lateral imbalances is rarely possible and that the imbalances tend to reoccur between trimming cycles. However, the practice of always

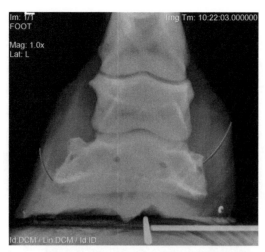

Fig. 6. A 0° dorsopalmar radiograph of an left front foot demonstrating proximal imbalance of the lateral aspect of the distal phalanx in combination with proximal displacement of the medial coronet in a horse with a medial quarter crack. The red lines denote the lateral and medial coronets.

attempting to correct the imbalances will help correct and limit hoof wall distortion. It is critical that uneven growth/imbalances are not ignored for successful long-term management. The fit of the shoe can be used to help improve the foot's platform. For example, in quarter crack cases whereby the medial or lateral hoof wall is excessively straight or rolls under, the corresponding branch of the shoe should be fit as full as practical to provide appropriate symmetry to the ground surface of the foot.

The correction/management of soft tissue displacements (proximally displaced coronets), if present, is accomplished by unloading or floating the displaced region. If the situation permits, the horse's shoes can be removed, the feet are trimmed such that the hoof wall at the heels and the frog are on the same plane, and the horse is then stood on a hard surface for 12 to 24 hours before trimming and shoeing. This practice can result in the affected side of the foot settling into a more acceptable conformation before completing the farriery. If a severe sheared heel hoof capsule distortion is present, the trimmed foot can be stood on some form of frog support and the foot placed in a soak bandage for 24 hours. This technique can produce a profound change in hoof shape in some cases. The specific farriery method used usually depends on personal preference. One method is to shoe the affected foot with a properly fit shoe with a rim pad (plastic or leather), minus the area of the pad that would contact the affected quarter and heel (**Fig. 7**A). This practice results in the region of the hoof with the displaced coronet being suspended (floated) approximately 0.125 to 0.25 in above the shoe. This suspension allows for the correction/improvement (settling) of the soft tissue displacement and also minimizes the external loads on the injured area. The gap between the shoe and the foot is filled with a small piece of weather stripping to prevent dirt/debris from accumulating in the floated region (see **Fig. 7**B, C). The solar surface of the foot is filled with a liquid urethane hoof packing material (Equi-Pak, Vettec Hoof Care Products, Oxnard, California) to help support the digit and minimize internal stresses on the crack. The urethane material is applied to ground level everywhere except in the region of the affected heel/quarter where it is only applied to shoe level. Applying the hoof packing in this manner maintains the float of the affected heel/quarter region.

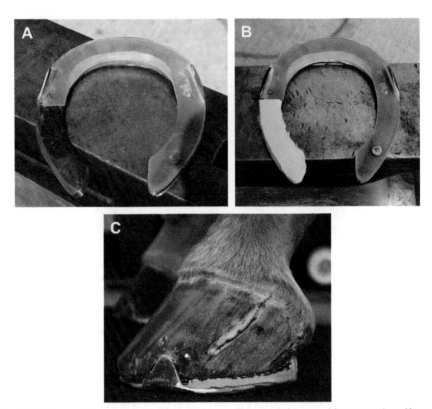

Fig. 7. (*A*) Shoe with a rim pad, minus the area of the pad that would contact the affected quarter and heel. (*B*) Weather stripping applied to prevent dirt accumulation. (*C*) Shoe applied. Note floating of the heel quarter and heel.

A second method involves a double-trimming technique. The affected foot is first trimmed appropriately as described earlier and then, before attaching the shoe, a second trim is performed under the proximally displaced quarter/heel.[10] The second trim begins at the ipsilateral toe and increases in depth toward the heel. The amount of heel that can be taken off in the second trim depends on the sole depth in the quarter/heel area. Ideally, the amount of heel removed corresponds to the amount of proximal displacement of the coronet. The foot is then shod with a symmetrically fitted wide web steel straight bar shoe, creating a space that resembles a wedge between the affected quarter/heel and the shoe (**Fig. 8**). If there is not enough sole depth under the affected heel for the second trim, the wall can be raised with a full leather pad. When a full pad is used, impression material (Equilox Pink, Equilox International, Pine Island, Minnesota) is placed beneath the pad to fill the frog sulci in the palmar section of the foot from the apex of the frog palmarly, except under the displaced heel. A third potential method used by one author (I.H.M.) on racehorses for floating the affected quarter/heel region is to trim the affected foot appropriately and then use a shoe that has a 2-component polyurethane rim pad affixed to it (Yasha Shoe, Tenderhoof Solutions, Ontario, Canada). The polyurethane in the heel area of the shoe is significantly softer than the polyurethane covering the rest of the shoe and, therefore, functionally unloads and floats the affected heel (**Fig. 9**).

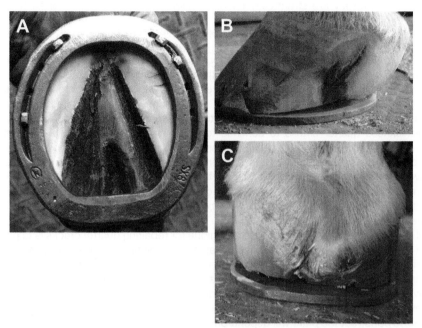

Fig. 8. (*A*) Steel straight bar shoe. Note the nails placed only in the toe area on the affected side (*B*) Lateral view showing hoof wall lowered from toe quarter to heel on second trim. Note space between the hoof wall and the shoe. (*C*) Palmar view showing the space below the sheared heel to allow the heel to settle distally.

If a horse with a full-thickness quarter crack is being taken out of work, the crack will not be repaired during the initial farriery. When the horse is presented for a subsequent reset, there should be significant new solid growth at the coronet above the defect. This growth would indicate that the initial farriery is effective in unloading the affected heel quarter. At this time, the crack can be repaired or allowed to grow out. If the crack is to be repaired, the defect should be debrided/explored with a motorized grinding tool or hoof knife, removing obviously undermined and diseased hoof wall. Exploration often reveals wall damage and undermining that exceeds initial visual appreciation. Care should be taken not to traumatize the dermis during debridement. No (or only occasional pinpoint) hemorrhage should occur during debridement. After debridement,

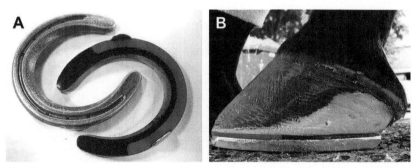

Fig. 9. (*A*) Yasha shoe. Note 2-component polyurethane rim pad. (*B*) Shoe applied functionally floating the heel region.

the crack defect should be treated with a topical disinfect/drying agent, such as 2% Tincture of Iodine or Thrush Buster (Delta Mustad Hoofcare, Lake Forest, Minnesota), at least once daily.

Ideally, horses with full-thickness quarter cracks should be taken out of work and allowed time for the inflammation to resolve, the dermal portions of the crack to heal, existing hoof distortions and soft tissue displacements to be corrected/improved, and the cracks to begin to be replaced by new wall before they are repaired. However, veterinarians and farriers often encounter situations when it is important for horses with full-thickness quarter cracks to continue to train and compete. In these cases, the repair/stabilization of the crack is often necessary before hoof distortions and soft tissue displacements can be corrected and sometimes before the dermal portions of the crack have healed/dried out sufficiently. Several techniques exist for repairing and allowing continued treatment of the crack in these cases. Fully addressing the hoof distortion and soft tissue displacement issues should be emphasized as soon as the horse can be taken out of work.

The first author's (R.S.P.) preferred technique for repairing quarter cracks is to plate the crack with a composite of polymethylmethacrylate adhesive (Equilox, Equilox International, Pine Island, Minnesota) and a polymeric fabric (Fig. 10). Before plating the crack, the hoof wall must be prepared to accept the adhesive (cleaned/sanded) and povidone iodine ointment (or another similar substance) applied into the crack bed to prevent the adhesive from entering the crack. The type and number of layers of fabric used to construct the plate will depend on the anticipated strength needed. For most cracks, 3 layers of polymethylmethacrylate saturated polyester/vectran fabric (Sound Horse Technologies, Unionville, Pennsylvania) provide sufficient strength. The plate should extend from the coronet to the distal surface of the hoof wall and at least 1.5 in dorsal and palmar from the edges of the crack. Each side of the polyester/vectran fabric is saturated with adhesive. The layers are then stacked and pressed together with a roller to expel excess adhesive. The plate is applied and allowed to cure with the foot unloaded so that the crack is stabilized in a neutral position. Small holes are then drilled proximally and distally through the repair into the crack defect to vent the crack or to allow continued treatment beneath the repair. The repair should be completely removed and reapplied (from the distal wall to the coronet) at least every other shoeing to minimize localized stress at the top of the repair. Complete reconstruction of the crack (filling the crack bed with adhesive as well as plating over the defect) may eventually be performed but only after the crack bed is completely dry. In many horses, a residual defect will remain apparent after the crack has grown out. This defect is manifested by a faint line or a slight inversion of the wall in the area of the previous crack and may represent permanent injury to the germinal tissues of the hoof wall as

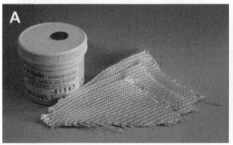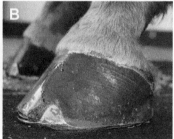

Fig. 10. (A) Polymethylmethacrylate adhesive and polymeric fabric. (B) Quarter crack plated with a polymethylmethacrylate adhesive and polymeric fabric composite.

a result of the original crack. In these cases, it is recommended to maintain the horse with a polymethylmethacrylate/polymeric fabric plate over the affected area whenever the horse is in training to reduce the risk of repeated cracks.

The second and third authors' (S.E.O. and I.M.) preferred technique for stabilizing quarter cracks involves inserting an implant comprising stainless steel wires first and then reinforcing the wires with a patch consisting of a mix of fiberglass strands and polymethylmethacrylate adhesive (**Fig. 11**).[11,12] Two sets of paired holes (0.25 in apart) are drilled perpendicular to the crack defect on each side of the crack, beginning at least 0.5 in from the margin of the defect and ending in the crack defect across from each other. The drilling is performed using a Dremel tool (Dremel, Racine, Wisconsin) and a 0.0469-in cobalt drill bit. A cobalt bit is used because it will not bend easily, which deters it from going in an undesired direction. Once the holes are drilled, the wire sets (Tenderhoof Solutions, Ontario, Canada) are inserted in palmar-to-dorsal and dorsal-to-palmar directions into the crack defect. The wires are then pulled tight and bent outwards. The wires go through steel tabs that lie against the hoof wall so that they will not pull through the wall. A drain is then created by placing a small amount of medicated putty (Keratex Hoof Putty, Keratex, Wiltshire, United Kingdom) into the crack bed and then pressing a thin piece of tubing or plastic string into the putty that exits at the top and bottom of the crack. The ends of the opposing wires are then joined together and twisted until resistance is felt. The horse should not show discomfort caused by overtightening of the wires. The excess wire is cut off at the top of the twist. Polymethylmethacrylate adhesive mixed with strands of fiberglass (Equilox, Equilox International, Pine Island, Minnesota) is then applied over the wires onto the hoof wall. It is thought that the composite mixed with strands of fiberglass add strength to the repair and provides better adhesion to the hoof wall. Care must be taken that the composite patch does not extend beyond the distal margin of the hoof wall to prevent this section of the hoof from being unloaded. On completion of the cure cycle, the drain is removed, allowing for continued treatment beneath the repair if necessary.

MANAGEMENT OF TOE CRACKS

In horses with toe cracks associated with long-toe, low-heel conformation, a radiographic evaluation often displays divergence of the distal dorsal hoof wall from the dorsal surface of the distal phalanx, excessive digital breakover, and a flat to negative distal phalanx palmar angle (**Fig. 12**A). The management of full-thickness toe cracks in

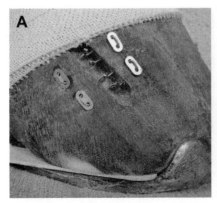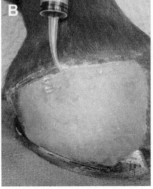

Fig. 11. (*A*) Quarter crack repair using stainless steel wires (implant). (*B*) Completed repair. Note the opening dorsally that can be used to flush interior of repair if necessary.

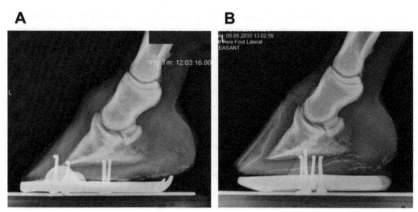

Fig. 12. (A) Lateromedial radiograph of a horse suffering from a full-thickness toe crack. (B) Proper trim and shoe fit of same foot.

horses with this type of conformation begins with trimming the feet using the guidelines outlined earlier.[10] The dorsal surface of the hoof wall should be dressed back to align with the dorsal surface of the distal phalanx. The feet should be shod with some form of enhanced breakover to reduce leverage on the toe. The shoes should also be fit to provide as much palmar support as practical to improve the foot's base of support and to encourage more appropriate hoof growth (see **Fig. 12**B).

In horses with toe cracks associated with an upright or clubfoot hoof conformation, the feet should be trimmed to establish parallel hoof-pastern axes and to shift the load away from the toe and onto the palmar section of the foot. This process can be accomplished by beginning the trim in the middle of the foot and trimming the foot in a tapered fashion toward the heels, which will create 2 planes on the ground surface of the foot. Any concavity in the dorsal hoof wall should be backed up from the dorsal surface. The feet should be shod with appropriately fit shoes with ample breakover created in the toe of the shoe. Care should be taken to prevent excess shoe pressure in the toe region.

The stabilization of toe cracks can be accomplished via several techniques. The first author (R.S.P.) prefers to stabilize toe cracks with polymethylmethacrylate adhesive saturated polymeric fabric plates (**Fig. 13**) using the same technique and principles

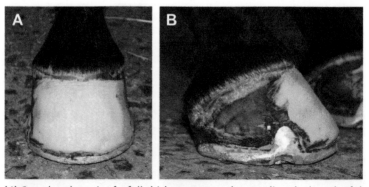

Fig. 13. (A) Completed repair of a full-thickness toe crack extending the length of the dorsal hoof wall using polymethylmethacrylate adhesive and polymeric fabric composite (B) Lateral view.

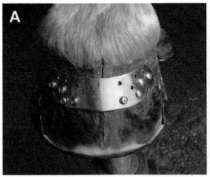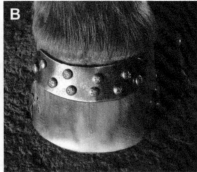

Fig. 14. (*A*) Toe crack repaired with a metal plate and screws. Note the plate is shaped to reflect the contour of the coronary band. (*B*) Same repair technique using a metal plate.

as described for quarter crack repair. Further stabilization of the foot (minimizing internal movement of the digit) is achieved by the use of some type of support shoe or heel plate shoe with impression material or via polyurethane sole support materials (EquiPak, Vettec Hoof Care Products, Oxnard, California). The second author (S.E.O.) prefers to stabilize toe cracks with a metal plate that bridges the crack and that is anchored on each side of the crack with screws. A lightweight, approximately 3×8 cm metal plate (steel, aluminum, or brass) is used. A 0.1406-in drill bit is used to make as many holes in the plate as necessary, with the holes positioned at least 0.5 cm apart and away from the crack. The plate is bent to conform to the contour of the coronary band and the curvature of the hoof wall and is positioned approximately 1 cm distal to the coronary band. The plate is applied with #6 0.375-in or smaller (depending on the thickness of the hoof wall) sheet metal screws and a screwdriver. At least 4 screws should be placed on each side of the crack for a secure application (**Fig. 14**). It is extremely important to attach the plate with the foot off of the ground or in the unloaded position. This placement ensures that the defect is affixed in the open position allowing better alignment and reducing any compression on the dermal papillae producing horn tubules.

SUMMARY

Quarter and toe cracks that result in the loss of the structural integrity of the hoof wall are not uncommon and usually manifest in lameness. From the perspective of pathogenesis and stabilization, these cracks should be thought of as wall fractures. From the perspective of healing, the cracks can only be eliminated by new, stable growth. Successful management involves identifying and addressing the underlying causes, stabilization of the foot, and committed follow-up to prevent reoccurrence.

REFERENCES

1. Davies HM, Philip C. Anatomy and physiology of the equine digit. In: Floyd AE, Mannsmann RA, editors. Equine podiatry. Philadelphia: Saunders Elsevier; 2007. p. 1–24.
2. Reilly JD, Collins SN, Cope BC, et al. Tubule density of the stratum medium of horse hoof. Equine Vet J Suppl 1998;26:4–9.
3. Bertram JE, Gosline JM. Fracture toughness design in horse hoof keratin. J Exp Biol 1986;125:29–47.

4. Kapasi MA, Gosline JM. Design complexity and fracture control in the equine hoof wall. J Exp Biol 1997;200:1639–59.
5. Reilly JD, Cottrell DF, Martin RJ, et al. Tubule density in the equine horn. Biomimetics 1996;4:23–35.
6. Davies HM, Philip C, Merritt JS. Functional anatomy of the equine digit: determining function from structure. In: Floyd AE, Mannsmann RA, editors. Equine podiatry. Philadelphia: Saunders Elsevier; 2007. p. 25–41.
7. Davies HM, Merritt JS, Thomason JJ. Biomechanics of the equine foot. In: Floyd AE, Mannsmann RA, editors. Equine podiatry. Philadelphia: Saunders Elsevier; 2007. p. 42–56.
8. Parks AH. The Foot and shoeing – foot balance, conformation, and lameness. In: Ross MW, Dyson SJ, editors. Diagnosis and management of lameness in the horse. 2nd edition. St Louis (MO): Elsevier Saunders; 2011. p. 282–93.
9. O'Grady SE. Foot care and farriery – basic foot care. In: Baxter GM, editor. Adams and Stashak's lameness in horses. 6th edition. West Sussex (United Kingdom): Wiley – Blackwell; 2011. p. 1179–98.
10. O'Grady SE, Castelijins HH. Sheared heels and the correlation to spontaneous quarter cracks. Equine Vet Educ 2011;23(5):262–9.
11. McKinlay I. Repairing quarter cracks and managing wall separations. In: Proceedings. Focus on the equine foot, American Association of Equine Practitioners. Lexington (KY) 2009. p. 175–80.
12. McKinlay I. Quarter crack repair educational video. On: Tenderhoof Solutions website. Available at: www.tenderhoof.com/. Accessed September 15, 2011.

Nonseptic Diseases Associated with the Hoof Complex

Keratoma, White Line Disease, Canker, and Neoplasia

W. Rich Redding, DVM, MS[a,*], Stephen E. O'Grady, DVM, MRCVS, APF[b]

KEYWORDS

• Hoof • White line disease • Hoof wall separation • Keratoma • Canker

KEY POINTS

- Keratoma is an uncommon cause of lameness unless associated with an infection; the treatment of choice is surgical removal of the keratoma, which is accomplished by dissection through the sole wall junction or by removal of the hoof wall over the mass.
- White line disease is a keratolytic process that occurs on the solar surface of the hoof, which is characterized by a progressive separation of the inner zone of the hoof wall. Successful treatment is twofold: correcting any predisposing causes and the application of the appropriate therapeutic farriery combined with resection of the affected hoof wall.
- Equine canker is as an infectious process that results in the development of a chronic, hypertrophic moist pododermatitis of the frog and the adjacent horn-producing structures.
- Neoplasia involving the equine foot is rare; of the few cases reported in the literature, melanoma is the most common type of neoplasm.

KERATOMA

Keratoma is a benign, keratin-containing soft-tissue mass that develops between the hoof wall and the distal phalanx (P3). Keratomas are thought to originate from the epidermal horn-producing cells of either the coronary or solar corium, although these lesions have not been extensively studied histologically.[1] Keratomas have been described as having an outer epidermal layer and a core of dense, laminated keratin, with no evidence of inflammatory infiltrate.[1] The lack of consistent histologic evaluation makes it difficult to determine a common etiology. Previous trauma or chronic irritation has been proposed as possible causes.

Keratomas act as space-occupying masses within the hoof capsule. Because they are usually located within the epidermal lamellae or the solar corium on the inner aspect of the hoof wall and exert pressure on P3, an area of bone resorption can be

[a] Department of Clinical Sciences, College of Veterinary Medicine, North Carolina State University, Raleigh, NC 27606, USA; [b] Northern Virginia Equine, PO Box 746, Marshall, VA 20116, USA
* Corresponding author.
E-mail address: rich_redding@ncsu.edu

Vet Clin Equine 28 (2012) 407–421
http://dx.doi.org/10.1016/j.cveq.2012.06.006
0749-0739/12/$ – see front matter © 2012 Elsevier Inc. All rights reserved.

seen radiographically in most cases, most often at the toe, but can be located anywhere around the perimeter of the distal phalanx.[2–5] In some cases, a submural keratoma extends to the solar surface of the foot, where it becomes evident as a distortion of the white line.

Clinical Findings

Keratoma is an uncommon cause of lameness unless associated with an infection. Clinical signs are variable, and may be related to the size and location of the keratoma. The keratoma can be located in the sole, under the hoof wall, and above the coronet. The lameness can be mild to moderate, depending on the degree of impingement on the sensitive dermal tissue. Severe lameness may be caused by disruption of normal hoof architecture, with subsequent abscess formation. If there is a history of recurrent abscesses localized to the same area, a keratoma should be suspected. The lameness may become progressively worse as the keratoma grows in size, increasing pressure on the sensitive lamellae.

Keratomas can change the shape of the coronary band (ie, create a bulge) in the affected area and, in more advanced cases, in the overlying hoof wall. In keratomas that extend down to the bearing surface of the hoof wall, thoroughly cleaning the sole may demonstrate an island of horn 1 to 2 cm in diameter in the white line, and deviation of the white line at that location toward the center of the foot (**Fig. 1**).

Diagnosis

The degree of lameness is often variable, and there will generally be a focal response to hoof testers. Unilateral palmar digital nerve block typically improves the lameness associated with a keratoma at the quarters, but it may be necessary to perform a basi-sesamoid (abaxial) bilateral nerve block to improve the lameness if the keratoma is located in the toe region. Radiographic examination often demonstrates a smoothly

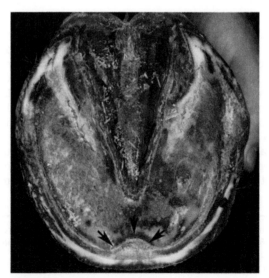

Fig. 1. In keratomas that extend down to the bearing surface of the hoof wall, thoroughly cleaning the sole may demonstrate an island of horn 1 to 2 cm diameter in the white line, and deviation of the white line at that location toward the center of the foot.

demarcated radiolucent defect in the solar margin of P3. Standard 65° dorsopalmar views are useful to identify this bony change (**Fig. 2**). Differential diagnoses include septic or nonseptic pedal osteitis, osseous cyst-like lesions, and benign or malignant neoplasms.

If a keratoma is suspected but there are no supporting radiographic findings, nuclear scintigraphy may be helpful, as active bone remodeling will be apparent as increased radionuclide uptake. Diagnostic ultrasonography can also be helpful in identifying keratomas at the coronary band.[4]

Treatment

The treatment of choice is surgical removal of the keratoma, which is accomplished by removal of the hoof wall over the mass. Historically a full-length strip of hoof wall over the keratoma is removed. However, removing this much of the wall can create excessive instability in the hoof wall and prolong convalescence.

If the keratoma can be isolated to a specific area by the use of radiography, computed tomography, or magnetic resonance imaging, the hoof wall can be removed at that site, allowing access to the mass for removal. Removal of the overlying horn can be accomplished using a Dremel tool or a trephine. If more hoof wall needs to be removed, the Dremel tool can be used to access and remove the entire keratoma mass. In many cases, the keratoma can be accessed and removed from the solar surface of the foot following the tract dorsally (**Fig. 3**).

Management of the hoof wall defect is as described for any wound to the foot. Stability can be increased by the use of a bar shoe with clips. Once adequate keratinization of the defect has occurred, more stability can be provided by reconstruction of the hoof wall with composite material/adhesives.

WHITE LINE DISEASE

White line disease (WLD) can be described as a keratolytic process on the solar surface of the hoof, which is characterized by a progressive separation of the inner zone of the hoof wall.[6–13] The separation occurs in the nonpigmented horn at the

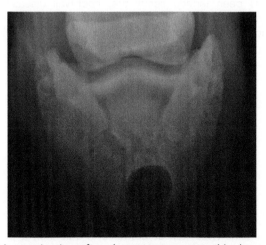

Fig. 2. Radiographic examination often demonstrates a smoothly demarcated radiolucent defect in the solar margin of P3. Standard 65° dorsopalmar views are useful to identify this bony change.

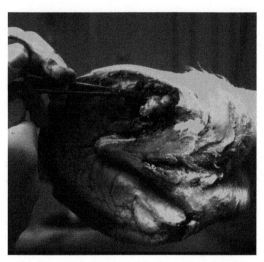

Fig. 3. In many cases, the keratoma can be accessed and removed from the solar surface of the foot following the tract dorsally. Removal of the overlying horn can be accomplished using a Dremel tool or a trephine. If more hoof wall needs to be removed, the Dremel tool can be used to access and remove the entire keratoma mass.

junction between the stratum medium and the stratum internum (**Fig. 4**A, B). A separation in the hoof wall is considered to be a delaminating process that could potentially originate from genetics, mechanical stress, environmental conditions affecting the inner hoof wall attachment, and possibly some toxicity such as selenium. In fact, the cause of hoof-wall separations remains speculative. Hoof -all separation can originate at the toe, the quarter, and/or the heel, and appears to be invaded by opportunistic bacteria/fungi. These organisms lead to infections that can progresses to varying heights and configurations proximally toward the coronet. This disease process always occurs secondary to a hoof-wall separation.

The disease has been termed seedy toe, hoof-wall disease, yeast infection, Candida, and onychomycosis. However, mycotic disease originates in the nail bed of the human and the dog, in contrast to WLD in the horse where the infection

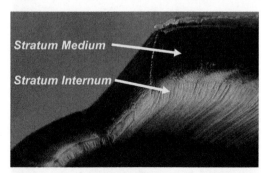

Fig. 4. White line disease (WLD) can be described as a keratolytic process on the solar surface of the hoof, which is characterized by a progressive separation of the inner zone of the hoof wall. The separation occurs in the nonpigmented horn at the junction between the stratum medium and the stratum internum.

originates at the solar surface of the hoof and migrates proximally toward the coronet. WLD in the horse can approach the coronet but never invades it. Keratophilic fungi are often isolated from affected areas of the hoof wall; however, in many cases of WLD, the pathogens cultured are purely bacterial or are a mix of bacterial and fungal organisms.

Anatomy of the Hoof Wall

A review of the hoof-wall anatomy may be helpful in understanding the location on the solar surface of the hoof where hoof-wall separations occur.

The hoof wall consists of 3 layers:

- The stratum externum (external layer)
- The stratum medium (middle layer)
- The stratum internum (inner layer)

The stratum externum (periople) arises from the perioplic epidermis and forms the thin outer layer of keratinized cells that give the wall its smooth, glossy appearance. The stratum medium, which arises from the coronary epidermis, forms the bulk of the hoof wall and is the densest part of the horny wall. It consists of cornified epidermal cells arranged in parallel horny tubules surrounded by intertubular horn, which grows distally from the coronary groove to the basal border. In all hooves it is always nonpigmented in the deepest inner layer. The stratum internum (epidermal lamellae) arises from the lamellar epidermis, is nonpigmented, and when combined with the dermal lamellae is responsible for attaching the hoof wall to the distal phalanx. Distally at the sole-wall junction, the dermal lamellae end in terminal papillae. The terminal papillae produce terminal tubules surrounded by intertubular horn that fills the spaces between the nonpigmented epidermal lamellae laminae. This association forms the bond between the hoof wall and the sole, known as the white line or white zone.[10] When observed from the solar surface, this white line or zona alba is actually yellow in color and has a plastic consistency when compared with the dorsal hoof wall (**Fig. 5**).

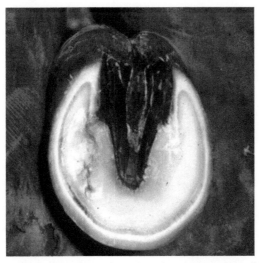

Fig. 5. When observed from the solar surface, this white line or zona alba is actually yellow in color and has a plastic consistency when compared with the dorsal hoof wall.

Etiology

WLD can affect a horse of any age, sex, or breed. One or multiple feet may be involved, and the affected horses can be barefoot or shod. One or multiple horses on the same farm may be affected. The problem occurs worldwide. Multiple causes of WLD have been proposed, but none have been proved. Among the speculative causes are excessive moisture and excessively dryness that may initiate and perpetuate separations allowing invasion of pathogens, poor hygiene, and infectious organisms (bacteria, fungi, or a combination of both). The fact that WLD can be resolved with thorough debridement alone further detracts from infection as a primary cause.[11] Mechanical stress placed on the inner part of the hoof wall may predispose to a separation and appears to be the logical cause. Forms of mechanical stress would include excessive toe length and various hoof-capsule distortions such as long toe-under run heel, clubfoot, or sheared heels.

Clinical Signs

WLD offers no threat to the soundness of the horse until damage is sufficient to allow mechanical loss of the attachment between the external lamellae and the inner hoof wall, resulting in displacement of the distal phalanx (P3) in a distal direction (rotation and/or sinking). Pain may also result from solar contusion and increased stress in the lamellae at the margins of large areas of separations. In the early stages of WLD, the only noticeable change seen on the solar surface of the foot is a small powdery area located just abaxial to the sole/wall junction (white line). This area may remain localized or it may progress to involve a larger area of the hoof wall. If the separation becomes more extensive and extends into a quarter, a concavity ("dish") can be seen forming along the unaffected side of the hoof and a bulge will be present on the ipsilateral side at the proximal extent of the separation at the coronary band (**Fig. 6**). This situation arises from extensive loss of epidermal lamellae on the side with the separation, which results in a loss of equilibrium between the lateral and medial side of the foot, causing the hoof capsule to shift toward the unaffected side of the foot. There may be a decrease in hoof-wall growth, poor consistency of the hoof wall, and a hollow sound noted when the outer hoof wall is hit with a hammer. Often the disease goes undetected until the horse begins to show signs of lameness.

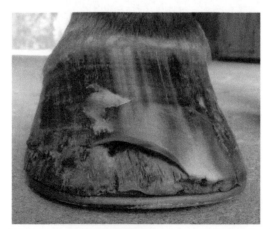

Fig. 6. A concavity ("dish") can be seen forming along one side of the hoof, and a bulge will be present on the opposite side directly above the affected area at the coronary band.

Diagnosis

Lameness may not be observed in the early stages. Hoof-tester examination does not always elicit a response. A thorough examination of the solar surface of the hoof wall will generally provide a diagnosis. On the solar surface of the hoof, often at the toe, in the early stages of the disease the sole-wall junction (white line) will be wider, softer, and may have a chalky texture. As the disease progresses, a hoof-wall separation will deepen and become evident. Exploring the inner hoof wall, which lies dorsal to the sole-wall junction, will generally reveal a separation filled with white/gray, powdery horn material. Further exploration with a blunt probe will give the depth, direction, and extent of the separation. There may be a black serous drainage from the separation depending on the moisture content of the foot.[11] If lameness is present, a thorough lameness examination should be performed, including diagnostic analgesia to localize and confirm the suspected area, followed by radiographs. With extensive hoof-wall damage, WLD accompanied by pain can mimic laminitis both clinically and radiographically.

Radiographs

Radiology can provide very important information and should be considered necessary for the appropriate diagnosis of WLD. Radiographic examination can be helpful in showing the extent of the hoof-wall separation and the degree of displacement of the distal phalanx within the hoof capsule. A farriery or podiatry study should be included as part of the radiographic examination, and should consist of a lateral to medial and dorsopalmar 0° views with the primary beam directed just above the solar surface of the foot. These views are important in outlining the location and extent of the WLD and separation of the hoof wall, and allow the clinician to differentiate between WLD and systemic laminitis (**Fig. 7**). Radiographically the separation in the lamellae will originate at the solar surface of the foot in WLD, whereas the lucency will originate in the dermal lamellae extending distally to the terminal laminar papillae in laminitis. Pedal osteitis may be noted in chronic cases of WLD. Finally, radiographs can be used as a guide for applying appropriate farriery.

Laboratory

Laboratory findings such as culture results have been unrewarding in directing treatment of this disease. Cultures have proved to be of little value because the samples taken from the separations are contaminated with dirt and opportunistic organisms.

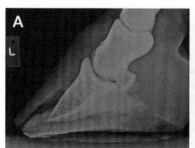
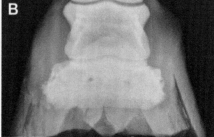

Fig. 7. A podiatry study should be included as part of the radiographic examination, and should consist of a lateral to medial (*A*) and dorsopalmar 0° (*B*) views directed just above the solar surface of the foot. These views are important in outlining the location and extent of the WLD and separation of the hoof wall, and allowing the clinician to differentiate between WLD and systemic laminitis.

Aerobic cultures usually reveal a mixed bacteria flora while anaerobic cultures are negative. Fungal cultures require a special medium and a prolonged time period to allow for adequate growth, with the most common fungal species recovered being *Pseudoallsheria*, *Scopulariopsis*, and *Aspergillus*. Furthermore, when bacteria and fungi are cultured together on the same culture plate, the fungi will quickly dominate the medium and become the predominant species.[12] A biopsy taken at the juncture between the normal and affected hoof wall shows a mixed population of microorganisms that will generally include coccobacilli, yeast organisms, and fungal spores. Inflammation in the laminar dermis will be seen deep to the affected area.[12]

Treatment

Successful treatment of WLD is twofold: it requires application of appropriate therapeutic farriery, or correction of inappropriate farriery combined with resection of the affected hoof wall. Farriery is directed at improving any existing hoof-capsule distortions as well as protecting and unloading the damaged section of the foot with the application of therapeutic shoeing. Resection disrupts the continuity and weight-bearing strength of the hoof wall, necessitating the application of some type of shoe to stabilize the hoof capsule and prevent the horse from using the sole for weight bearing. If the separation is determined to be extensive, a shoe should be designed and applied before the hoof wall is resected.

Farriery

The appropriate farriery should begin with the trim.[13] Trimming the foot should improve the foot conformation whenever possible. This action is generally accomplished by creating more ground surface on the solar surface of the foot by trimming the heels in a palmar/plantar direction, reducing the length of the toe, and being attentive to the medial-lateral orientation of the foot. In the early stage of the disease before extensive separation is present, the inner hoof wall dorsal to the sole-wall junction should be explored down to solid horn using a thin loop knife and then packed with a medicated putty (Component Cooler; RadioShack Corp, Fort Worth, TX) before attaching the shoe.

When hoof-wall resection is required, the authors consider it necessary that the horse have a therapeutic shoe applied and not be managed in the barefoot state. The type of horseshoe used and the method of attachment will depend on the extent of the damaged hoof wall. As the toe is involved in most cases of WLD, it is beneficial to move the breakover in a palmar/plantar direction. The ground surface of the foot is trimmed from the apex of the frog palmarly/plantarly, thus creating 2 planes on the solar surface of the foot, which will redistribute the load from the dorsal area to the palmar/plantar section of the foot. The shoe is fitted such that a line drawn across the widest part of the foot will be in the middle of the shoe, and breakover is placed just dorsal to the distal phalanx in an attempt to further unload the dorsal hoof wall and remove the "moment arm" at the toe. This action will also stop the pinching effect that often occurs at the junction of normal hoof wall and the resection during the breakover phase of the stride.

If the resection is extensive and/or if rotation of the distal phalanx is present, some type of bar shoe, rail shoe, or a wooden shoe is used to stabilize the foot. If there is advanced displacement of the distal phalanx, some form of heel elevation may be necessary with the type of shoe that is selected. An alternative method would be to use a bar shoe or shoe that is open at the heels combined with some type of silastic material (Frank's Pharmacy, Ocala, FL) applied to the solar surface of the foot to redistribute the load. Attaching glue-on shoes to the ground surface of the foot is another useful method for shoeing the horse with WLD. This method is useful when there is limited hoof wall available for attaching the horseshoe with nails, and allows easy access to the resected section of the foot. The authors have not found the use of any type of boot to be advantageous in treating WLD, as a moist environment is created in the interior of the boot.

Resection
Complete hoof-wall resection (removal of outer hoof wall to expose diseased area) and debridement of all tracts and fissures in the affected area is necessary. The hoof wall is resected using any variety of tools such as a Dremel drill, half-round nippers, or a sharp loop knife. Debridement should be continued proximally and marginally until there is a solid attachment between the hoof wall and external lamellae. Further tracts and fissures are removed from the external lamellae using a Dremel tool with a drum sander **(Fig. 8)**. The veterinarian or farrier performing the resection should not reach blood during resection and debridement.

After thorough hoof-wall resection, the horse is placed on wood shavings or sawdust bedding, attempting to keep the feet dry. The resected area is left open to grow out. A wire brush is used daily by the owner to keep the resected area clean. Thorough exploration and debridement of any remaining tracts should take place at 2-week intervals. Thorough examination with the shoe removed is indicated at re-shoeing intervals of every 4 to 5 weeks.

The traditional approach of covering a resection with a composite should be discouraged. Composite repair should only be considered only after all tracts are resolved, and should only be used in selected cases where the client is unable to treat the resected area and where cosmetics are a necessity. If a composite repair is elected, an interface with a material such as modeling clay should be placed between the composite and the surface of the epidermal lamellae. When the composite is placed directly on the epidermal lamellae, it may hide and/or foster infection under the repair and can weaken surrounding normal hoof wall, which can encourage reinfection.

Medical treatment
There has been a plethora of topical medications described for treating WLD either with or without a hoof-wall resection, but as yet there is no scientific proof as to their efficacy. Furthermore, medical treatment in any form is of no value without resection of the affected hoof wall. Medical treatment may not be necessary in most cases, as

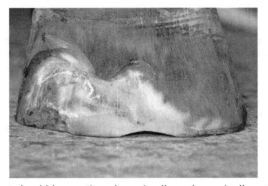

Fig. 8. Debridement should be continued proximally and marginally until there is a solid attachment between the hoof wall and external lamellae by using a Dremel tool with a drum sander.

debridement alone appears to be sufficient. Disinfectants/astringents such as methiolate or 2% iodine act as a good disinfectant and drying agent, but may have more benefit as a dye marker to outline the remaining tracts. The dye marker will serve as a visual aid in outlining the remaining tracts at subsequent examinations and as a guide during debridement. Either preparation should be applied weekly, as excessive applications make the exposed epidermal lamina excessively hard.

Aftercare

A change in the horse's environment is important for management of WLD. The feet should be kept as dry as possible throughout the recovery period. When the horse is confined to a stall, it should be placed on a wood shavings or sawdust-type bedding while keeping the bedding clean and dry. Limited turnout in heavy rain or wet weather will decrease excess moisture in the foot. Turnout can be delayed in the morning until the sun dries the dew from the pasture. A shoeing schedule should be maintained at 4-week intervals.

Treatment requires a commitment from the owner to provide a continuous treatment schedule to eliminate all signs of disease. The extent of the damage will determine the amount of time required for the treatment process. However, it is not always necessary for the horse to be out of work for all of this period. The amount of exercise permissible while treating WLD is dependent on the extent of the damage and the presence of sufficient hoof wall necessary for weight bearing. It has always been the authors' rule that if the resection extends beyond a point halfway up the hoof capsule when measured from the ground to the coronet, the horse should be taken out of work.

Prevention

Prevention of WLD is difficult because the exact cause is unknown. Discussing the problem with the farrier and having him or her examine each foot when the horse is shod is extremely important. Any abnormal area regardless of size that involves the sole/wall junction should be explored and debrided down to solid horn. Any cavity created by debridement can be filled with medicated putty before being covered with a shoe. Proper physiologic trimming and shoeing is essential for creating a strong sole/wall junction that prevents separations and offers protection against migrating organisms.[13] It is equally important to carefully monitor horses that have previously had WLD. A year or two after WLD has been treated and resolved, it can suddenly reappear in some horses that had developed normal-appearing hoof walls.

EQUINE CANKER

Equine canker is described as an infectious process that results in the development of a chronic hypertrophy of the horn-producing tissues.[14–18] Canker generally originates in the frog or associated sulci and often remains focal, but has the capacity to become diffuse and invade the adjacent sole, bars, and hoof wall. Canker can occur in one foot or multiple feet. The disease is commonly seen in draft breeds but can affect any breed. The etiology of canker remains elusive, but wet environmental or moist unhygienic conditions have traditionally been thought to act as a stimulus. However, canker is commonly seen in horses that are well cared for and in horses that receive regular hoof care. Until recently, no one treatment has been consistently effective in treating this disease, and the prognosis has always been guarded.

Clinical Signs

Canker can be and often is mistaken for thrush in the early stages of the disease, as both generally originate in the frog. However, thrush is typically limited to the lateral and medial sulci or the base of the frog if a fissure is present, whereas canker invades the horn of the frog anywhere throughout its structure. Canker commonly presents with a proliferation of tissue whereas thrush presents as a loss of tissue. If canker is noticed in the early stages, it may present as a small focal area of what appears to be granulation tissue in the frog that bleeds easily when abraded. If left untreated, the disease will become diffuse and involve the frog, bars, sole, and stratum medium of the hoof wall in the palmar/plantar aspect of the foot. Canker in the advanced stage is characterized by numerous small finger-like papillae of soft off-white material that resembles a cauli-flower-like appearance (**Fig. 9**).[14–17] The condition is frequently but not always accompanied by a foul odor, and is covered with a caseous white exudate that resembles cottage cheese. The characteristic putrid odor will be absent if the animal has been treated with various topical medications before the clinician's examination. The affected tissue will bleed easily when abraded and may be extremely painful when touched. Varying degrees of lameness will be present, depending on the extent and depth of the infection.

Diagnosis

A presumptive diagnosis of canker is based on the gross appearance of the affected horny tissue along with a fetid odor; however, a definitive diagnosis may only be confirmed with a biopsy. The biopsy sample should include both normal and abnormal tissue.[14] Histologically the lesion is read as a chronic, hypertrophic, moist pododermatitis of the frog. Cultures are unrewarding, as they typically produce an assortment of opportunistic environmental organisms such as *Bacteroides* spp and *Fusobacterium necrophorum*.[16]

Treatment

The authors' preferred treatment consists of thorough, careful debridement of the affected tissue, followed by cryotherapy and a regimen of topical therapy applied daily

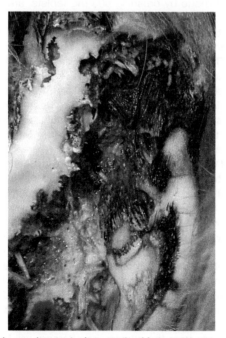

Fig. 9. Canker in the advanced stage is characterized by numerous small finger-like papillae of soft off-white material that resembles a cauliflower-like appearance.

and continued until the disease is resolved. To debride the affected tissue, the horse can be placed under general anesthesia, or regional anesthesia can be used with the horse standing. An often ignored and very important aspect of treatment is to trim the horse's foot before surgery. The foot is trimmed to remove all loose exfoliating sole, and the heels are trimmed such that the hoof wall at the heels and the frog are on the same plane. The frog should not be recessed between the heels of the hoof wall at the beginning of treatment. The use of a tourniquet such as an Esmarch bandage, placed over the vessels at the fetlock, is essential to create a bloodless field so that the demarcation between normal and diseased tissue can be seen during debridement. All abnormal tissue is removed down to normal corium. A clear demarcation such as a color change and numerous pinpoint hemorrhages, which are the dermal papillae, will be observed between normal and abnormal tissue. Debridement needs to be thorough and wide rather than aggressive and deep, which often leads to removal of the dermal tissue under the lesion that is necessary for regrowth and cornification. It is important not to remove excessive corium, as this will retard cornification following surgery and may decrease the quality and depth of new horn being produced. It may be helpful to remove 1 to 2 cm of normal tissue around the wound margins to ensure that all abnormal tissue is removed. Debridement can be performed using a sharp loop knife and a #12 scalpel blade. The debridement is followed by cryotherapy to freeze the area that has been debrided. Liquid nitrogen is commonly used for this purpose, but another practical method is to freeze the debrided area with a coolant spray (Component Cooler; RadioShack Corp) that is available for electrical circuits. The area of the foot that has been debrided will be soft and pliable. The affected area is frozen until the tissue becomes hard (known as a hard freeze) then is allowed to thaw, and then the freeze is repeated once more. Gauze 4 × 4 sponges moistened in a solution of 10% benzoyl peroxide in acetone (Frank's Pharmacy), sprinkled with metronidazole powder made by crushing 500-mg tablets, are then placed over the debrided site. In large defects, especially where the debrided tissue is recessed below the ground surface of the hoof wall, a dental impression material (Equilox Pink; Equilox International, Pine Island, MN) is used to form an insert to fit over the surgical site in the bottom of the foot. The impression material will ensure contact of the medication against the tissue in the depths of the wound while exerting mild pressure to minimize the production of exuberant granulation tissue. This mild pressure also appears to promote physiologic function of the frog (**Fig. 10**). The impression material should not extend below the solar surface of the hoof wall, as this will create excess pressure and discomfort. The foot is then bandaged with a dry bandage. The bandage is changed daily or at least every second day, the affected area is cleaned with an antiseptic solution, rinsed with saline, dried with a paper towel, and the topical medication reapplied. It is crucial to keep the animal in a dry environment. A shoe with a treatment plate has been recommended, but the authors consider it difficult to keep the foot as dry as necessary with this method until full cornification is present. Focal reoccurrences may be managed with the horse standing with light debridement followed by cryotherapy. The use of systemic antibiotics such as chloramphenicol or oxytetracycline has been advocated, but the authors question this practice because most cases resolve with local treatment only. A recent scientific paper describes the adjunctive use of systemic prednisolone at a dose of 1 mg/kg every 24 hours for 7 days, 0.5 mg/kg every 24 hours for 7 days, and then 0.25 mg/kg every 24 hours for 7 days[18] during the treatment phase of canker. The authors have used this approach as an adjunct to the treatment already discussed, and have found it to be beneficial. A commitment is necessary from the owners, as aftercare will be labor intensive and may take several weeks, depending on the stage of the disease, until the affected

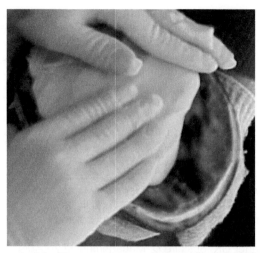

Fig. 10. Impression material will ensure contact of the medication against the tissue in the depths of the wound while exerting mild pressure to minimize the production of exuberant granulation tissue.

tissue is cornified. The combination of thorough surgical debridement/cryotherapy combined with topical application of benzoyl peroxide in acetone and metronidazole have yielded consistent predictable results.[14] Although the cause of canker remains obscure, there are several principles of therapy for this condition that the authors consider to be important. Thorough rather than aggressive debridement of the lesion is essential, along with methodical topical treatment. Cleaning the affected area daily with an antiseptic solution removes contaminating bacteria from the surface bacteria and provides an environment more conducive to wound healing. Ten-percent benzoyl peroxide in acetone is an excellent astringent and keeps the tissue dry. Cultures taken from lesions located on the solar surface of the foot generally yield anaerobic organisms, which make metronidazole a good antibiotic choice. Emphasis must be placed on keeping the surgical wound clean and dry until the defect begins to cornify. Owner compliance to perform daily foot care remains another essential element in the treatment of equine canker.

NEOPLASIA

Neoplasia involving the equine foot is rare. Of the few cases reported in the literature, melanoma is the most common type of neoplasm affecting the foot.[19–24] Squamous cell carcinoma and hemangioma involving the foot also have also been reported.[22]

Melanoma

Although this dermal tumor is commonly found in other parts of the horse's body, it occurs only rarely in the foot. Whereas most melanomas in the horse are benign or only minimally invasive, those reported to involve the foot invariably have been invasive (ie, malignant melanoma).[19–23] In cases of melanoma involving the foot, the presenting complaint was a draining tract or hoof-wall defect.[6–8] The clinical course was protracted, as long as 2 years in some cases. In each case, radiographic examination revealed marked osteolysis of P3. Thus, cases of recurrent foot abscess with marked osteolysis of P3 should be carefully evaluated for the possibility of not only keratomas but also neoplasia.[21–23]

Surgical biopsy of the tissue in the area of bone resorption is indicated in horses with this clinical appearance. Extensive removal of the abnormal tissue is the treatment of choice; however, it has not been curative in the few reported cases. All reported cases eventually resulted in euthanasia. Surgical resection, local chemotherapeutics, immunotherapeutics, or a combination of therapies may yield better results.[23]

REFERENCES

1. Hamir A, Kunz C, Evans L. Equine keratoma. J Vet Diagn Invest 1990;4:99–101.
2. Reeves MJ, Yovich JV, Turner AS. Miscellaneous conditions of the foot. Vet Clin North Am Equine Pract 1989;5:221–42.
3. Honnas CM, Dabareiner RM, McCauley BH. Hoof wall surgery in the horse: approaches to and underlying disorders. Vet Clin North Am Equine Pract 2003; 19:479–99.
4. Seahorn T, Sams A, Honnas C, et al. Ultrasonographic imaging of a keratoma in a horse. J Am Vet Med Assoc 1992;200:1973–4.
5. Chaffin MK, Carter GK, Sustaire D. Management of keratoma in a horse: a case report. J Equine Med Surg 1989;9:323–6.
6. O'Grady SE. White line disease—an update. Equine Vet Educ 2002;3:66–72.
7. Pleasant RS, O'Grady SE. White line disease. In: Robinson NE, editor. Current therapy in equine medicine. 6th edition. Philadelphia: W B Saunders; 2008. p. 528–32.
8. O'Grady SE. Farriery for common hoof problems. In: Baxter GM, editor. Adams and Stashak's lameness in horses. 6th edition. Ames (IA): Wiley-Blackwell; 2011. p. 1199–210.
9. Moyer W. Hoof wall defects: chronic hoof wall separations and hoof wall cracks. Vet Clin North Am Equine Pract 2003;19:463–77.
10. Parks AH. Form and function of the equine foot. Vet Clin North Am Equine Pract 2003;19:285–98.
11. O'Grady SE. How to manage white line disease. In: Proceedings of the 52nd Annual Convention of the American Association of Equine Practitioners. 2006.p. 520–5.
12. O'Grady SE. A fresh look at white line disease. Equine Vet Educ 2011;10:517–22.
13. Turner TA. White line disease. Equine Vet Educ 1998;4:73–6.
14. O'Grady SE. Guidelines for trimming the equine foot: a review. In: Proceedings of the 55th Annual Convention of the American Association of Equine Practitioners 2009;55. p. 218–25.
15. O'Grady SE. Madison JM. How to treat equine canker. In: Proceedings of the 50th Annual Convention of the American Association of Equine Practitioners 2004;50. p. 202–5.
16. Moyer WA, Colohan PT. Canker. In: Equine medicine & surgery. 5th edition. St Louis (MO): Mosby; 1999. p. 1544–6.
17. Turner TA. Treatment of equine canker. In: Proceedings of the 34th Annual Convention of the American Association of Equine Practitioners 1988. p. 307–10.
18. Wilson DG. Equine canker. In: Robinson NE, editor. Current therapy in equine medicine 4. Philadelphia: W.B. Saunders Co; 1997. p. 127–8.
19. Oosterlinck M, Deneut K, Dumoulin M, et al. Retrospective study of 30 horses with chronic proliferative pododermatitis (canker). Equine Vet Educ 2011;23:466–71.
20. Honnas CM, Liskey CC, Meagher DM, et al. Malignant melanoma in the foot of a horse. J Am Vet Med Assoc 1990;197:756–8.
21. Kunze DJ, Monticello TM, Jakob TP, et al. Malignant melanoma of the coronary band in a horse. J Am Vet Med Assoc 1986;188:297–8.

22. Floyd AE. Malignant melanoma in the foot of a bay horse. Eq Vet Educ American Edition 2003;5:379–81.
23. Berry CR, O'Brien TR, Pool RR. Squamous cell carcinoma in the hoof wall of a stallion. J Am Vet Med Assoc 1986;181:90–2.
24. Gelatt KJ, Neuwirth L, Hawkins DL, et al. Hemangioma of the distal phalanx in a colt. Vet Radiol Ultrasound 1990;37:275–80.

Septic Diseases Associated with the Hoof Complex

Abscesses, Punctures Wounds, and Infection of the Lateral Cartilage

W. Rich Redding, DVM, MS[a],*, Stephen E. O'Grady, DVM, MRCVS, APF[b]

KEYWORDS

- Hoof • Lameness • Hoof abscess • Puncture wound • Septic osteitis
- Lateral cartilage • Quittor

KEY POINTS

- Hoof abscesses are probably the most common cause of acute severe lameness in horses encountered by veterinarians and farriers.
- Most affected horses show sudden, severe (acute) lameness; the degree of lameness varies from being subtle in the early stages to non–weight bearing.
- There is still debate between the veterinary and farrier professions as to who should treat a hoof abscess and the best method in which to resolve the abscess.
- Puncture wounds to the sole of the foot can introduce bacteria and debris to the solar surface of the distal phalanx and frequently produce a fracture or a septic pedal osteitis.

INTRODUCTION

Anatomically, the foot comprises the hoof, the skin between the bulbs of the heels, and all the structures within. The hoof complex comprises the hoof capsule, sole, frog, digital cushion, ungual cartilages, and deep digital flexor tendon.[1] These biologic structures are susceptible to trauma and are prone to various disease processes, including infections (hoof abscesses, puncture wounds, and keratomas), white line disease, and canker. The equine foot is designed to perform numerous functions, including bearing the weight of the horse at all gaits, protecting the structures contained within the hoof capsule, absorbing concussion as the hoof strikes the ground, along with providing traction.[2] The unique interrelationship of the structures working in concert and the viscoelastic nature of the hoof capsule allow the hoof to perform these functions. The hoof wall, sole, frog, and bulbs of the heels compose the hoof capsule, which, through the unique continuous bond between its components, forms a casing

[a] Department of Clinical Sciences, College of Veterinary Medicine, North Carolina State University, Raleigh, NC 27606, USA; [b] Northern Virginia Equine, PO Box 746 Marshall, VA 20116, USA
* Corresponding author.
E-mail address: rich_redding@ncsu.edu

Vet Clin Equine 28 (2012) 423–440
http://dx.doi.org/10.1016/j.cveq.2012.06.004
0749-0739/12/$ – see front matter © 2012 Elsevier Inc. All rights reserved.

on the ground surface of the foot, which affords protection to the dermal and osseous structures enclosed within the capsule.[2] Furthermore, optimal protection is reliant on overall hoof health and a strong hoof capsule, which can be influenced by genetics, environment, exercise, and farriery practices.

The dermis or corium lines the inner surface of the hoof capsule and connects the hoof capsule to the underlying structures. The dermal tissue that seems most susceptible to injury is the laminar and solar corium. The bond or junction between the hoof wall and sole is especially important because it becomes susceptible to damage when subjected to the continuous repetitive stress of weight bearing. Damage here may allow a portal of entry for pathogens to invade the interior of the hoof capsule. Distally at the sole-wall junction, the dermal lamellae end in terminal papillae. These papillae are lined by stratum germinativum, which produces flexible horn tubules that are interspersed with intertubular horn that, between them, fill the spaces between the nonpigmented epidermal lamellae and the horny sole. This association forms the bond between the hoof wall and the sole known as the white line or zone. The sole-wall junction extends around the circumference of the solar surface of the foot and at the heels; it runs forward on the abaxial surface of the bars. Pathogens or debris that may lead to infection commonly penetrate the hoof capsule in 1 of 3 ways:

- A separation or defect in the hoof wall
- A fissure or tract in the sole-wall junction
- A puncture wound through the sole or the frog

A puncture wound could also include a misplaced horseshoe nail. This article describes the most current information and the most practical treatment of disease processes that occur within the hoof capsule, such as hoof abscesses, puncture wounds, and infection of the lateral cartilage. These diseases generally originate on the ground surface of the foot, penetrate the hoof capsule, and extend toward/into the dermal structures of the foot.

INFECTIONS WITHIN THE HOOF CAPSULE
Hoof Abscesses

Hoof abscesses are probably the most common cause of acute severe lameness in horses encountered by veterinarians and farriers. A hoof abscess can be defined as a localized accumulation of purulent exudate located between the germinal and keratinized layers of the epithelium, most commonly subsolar or submural.

MECHANISM

It may be easier to understand how to treat an abscess by a brief look at the mechanism by which an abscess forms. The cause of most abscesses is not specifically identifiable. At the time that they are diagnosed, many abscesses are associated with defects in the white line (**Fig. 1**).

Additionally, when an abscess is exposed for drainage, the deep side of the cavity usually comprises a thin layer of keratinized epidermis. These findings suggest that many abscesses form following microfracture or the formation of a similar defect in the white line or the immediately adjacent sole. The logical extension is that foreign material and bacteria are able to penetrate through the keratinized layer of the epidermis (stratum corneum). This penetration initiates an inflammatory response that is accompanied by the migration of white cells and fluid from the dermal vessels through the basement membrane and germinal layer of the epithelium to form the abscess. This process causes the separation of the germinal and cornified epithelium.

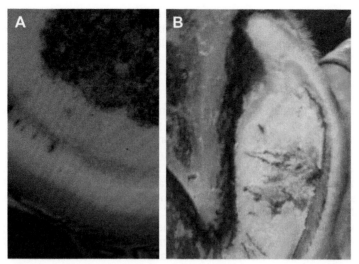

Fig. 1. (*A, B*) Foreign debris will gain entry and accumulate in a small separation or fissure located in the sole-wall junction anywhere around the perimeter of the foot including the abaxial surface of the bars adjacent to the sole (*B*).

The low compliance of the hoof capsule compared with the rest of the integument means that the pressure associated with the abscess increases rapidly, applying pressure on the underlying dermis. This pressure and the release of inflammatory mediators result in pain. Subsolar bruising is known to play a role in the development of some abscesses, namely, corns that have become septic. It is likely, therefore, that a subsolar bruise around the periphery of the foot is likely to potentiate the development of an abscess adjacent to the white line but how frequently this occurs is unknown. Abscesses that are not treated tend to expand and progress along the line of least resistance. In doing so, they cause progressive separation of the cornified and germinal epidermis and frequently breakout at the coronary band. Because simple abscesses are superficial to the epidermis, the repair of the defect once the infection has been eliminated is simply by proliferation and differentiation of the epidermal cells until the full thickness of the defect has been replaced.

Less commonly, an abscess may extend deep to the germinal layer of the epidermis to enter the dermis and underlying tissues. This extension causes necrosis of the underlying tissues. The healing process once the germinal layer of the dermis has been destroyed is different, and these wounds have to heal by the classical processes of inflammation and debridement followed by fibroplasia and epithelialization and the subsequent maturation.

CLINICAL SIGNS

Most affected horses show sudden severe (acute) lameness. The degree of lameness varies from being subtle in the early stages to non–weight bearing. The digital pulse felt at the level of the fetlock is typically increased (usually bounding), and the involved foot will be warmer than the opposite foot. With careful observation, unless the abscess is in the middle of the toe, the intensity of the digital pulse will be much stronger on the side of the foot where the infection is located. If the abscess is longstanding, there may be soft tissue swelling in the pastern up to or even above the fetlock on the side of the limb corresponding to the side of the foot where the abscess is located. The site of pain can be localized to a small focal area through the careful use of hoof testers. Sometimes with acute lameness, the pain will be noted over the foot with hoof testers; in this case, it is necessary to rule out laminitis, a severe bruise, or even a possible fracture of the distal phalanx (P3).

TREATMENT

There is still debate between the veterinary and farrier professions as to who should treat a hoof abscess and the best method in which to resolve the abscess. Considering that a walled off hoof abscess is an extension of the epidermis, it is the authors' opinion that the infection could be treated by either clinician. The most important aspect of treating a subsolar/submural hoof abscess is to establish drainage. The opening should be of sufficient size to allow drainage but not so extensive as to create further damage. When pain is localized with hoof testers, a small tract or fissure will commonly be found in the sole-wall junction. The wound or point of entry may not always be visible because some areas of the foot, such as the sole-wall junction, are somewhat elastic and tracts in this area tend to close. In this case, a suitable poultice should be applied to the foot daily in an attempt to soften the affected area and eventually a tract will become obvious.

When a tract or fissure is found, it can be followed/explored within the white line using a small, thin, loop knife, a 2-mm bone curette, or other suitable probe (**Fig. 2**). The tract is slowly followed until a gray/black exudate (pus) is released and the probe enters the belly of the abscess. At this point, the tract is open into the cavity of the abscess. A small opening is all that is necessary to obtain proper drainage (**Fig. 3**) and this can be determined by placing thumb pressure on the solar side of the tract and observing the expression of more exudates or a bubble forming at the opening of the track when pressure is applied. Care should be taken to avoid exposing any corium because it will invariably prolapse through the opening, preventing closure of the tract and possibly creating an ongoing source of pain. *Under no circumstances should an abscess be approached through the sole.*

The draining tract can be kept soft and drainage promoted in several ways. The authors will generally apply a medicated poultice (Animalintex 3M Animal Care Products, St Paul, Minnesota) for the first 24 to 48 hours. The poultice is immersed in hot

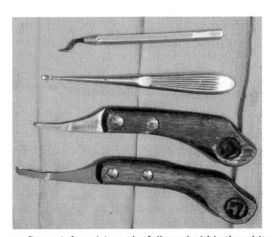

Fig. 2. When a tract or fissure is found, it can be followed within the white line using a small, thin loop knife, a 2-mm bone curette, or other suitable probe.

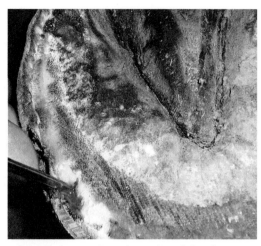

Fig. 3. At this point, the tract is open into the cavity of the abscess. A small opening is all that is necessary to obtain proper drainage.

water, placed on the foot, and attached with a roll of wide brown gauze, a cohesive bandage, and waterproof tape. The sheet version of this poultice is preferred rather than the poultice hoof pad that is distributed by the company. The whole foot, including the coronet, should be enveloped in the poultice. Another method to encourage drainage is to apply a soak bandage. Here layers of practical (pound) cotton are stacked together that will envelope the foot to form a heavy bandage. Magnesium sulfate (Epsom salts) is placed on the inner foot surface of the bandage and the bandage is attached to the foot as previously discussed. The bandage is now saturated with hot water and saturated periodically over the next 24 to 48 hours. Using either of these methods eliminates the need for continued foot soaking.

Ichthammol ointment, which is a coal tar derivative with mild antiseptic properties, has been described for treating skin disease in both humans and animals. The use of an ichthammol bandage for treating hoof abscesses, both before and after drainage, has become another traditional treatment among veterinarians and horse owners with reportedly good results. There are numerous commercial products marketed to treat foot abscesses but these products will only be helpful if they compliment the principles of drainage described previously.

Once drainage is established, the horse should show marked improvement within 24 hours. Once drainage has ceased, the hoof is kept bandaged with an appropriate antiseptic, such as Betadine (Betadine, Prodine Solution, First Priority, Inc, Elgin, Illinois) solution/ointment or 2% iodine applied over the tract until the wound is dry and sealed. At this point, the opening of the tract is filled with Keratex Hoof Putty (Keratex Medicated Hoof Putty, Brookville, Maryland), which keeps the affected area clean and prevents the accumulation of debris within the tract or wound. The shoe is replaced when the horse is completely sound.

Often, a painful tract can be located but drainage cannot be established at the sole-wall junction. In this case, the infection is deep and may have migrated under the sole or wall away from the sole-wall junction or white line. *Again, under no circumstances should an opening be created in the adjacent sole.* This infection seldom leads to the abscess and often leads to hemorrhage and may create a persistent, nonhealing wound with an increased potential for osteomyelitis of P3. Instead, a small channel can be created on the hoof wall side of the sole-wall junction using a small pair of half-round nippers. The channel is made in a proximal direction following the tract to the point where it meets the plane of the solar germinal epidermis at which point it courses toward the center of the sole. Drainage can usually be established using a small probe in a horizontal plane. Preferably, this is done at an early stage of the lameness before the infection ruptures at the coronet.

If left untreated, a hoof abscess will follow the path of least resistance along the outer margin of the dermal tissue and eventually rupture at the coronet forming a draining tract. Many horse owners actually consider this to be an acceptable practice and elect to wait for this to take place. This practice often extends the time the animal experiences severe pain. Rupture at the coronet also leads to a permanent scar under the hoof wall. This tract leading to the coronet may result in a prolonged recovery from the abscess, a chronic draining tract, repeated abscesses, and a full-thickness hoof wall crack. Every effort should be made to establish drainage on the solar surface of the foot before a rupture at the coronet.

INFECTION FROM A MISPLACED HORSESHOE NAIL

Deeper epidermal and dermal tissue can be inoculated by bacteria from a misplaced nail in 2 ways. The nail can be driven directly into the laminar corium. When the nail enters dermal tissue, the horse will generally show discomfort as the nail is driven into the foot and there will be hemorrhage present where the nail exits the outer hoof wall. Blood observed at the exit of the offending nail will alert the farrier of the misplaced nail. The blood also acts as a physiologic rinse to dilute or eliminate bacterial contamination. Removing the nail and applying an appropriate antiseptic will usually prevent infection. Another scenario that occurs frequently is when the horse shows discomfort while the farrier is driving a nail, indicating that the nail is invading sensitive tissue. Often, the farrier will remove the nail, place it in another spot/direction, and again drive it into the foot. However, when this scenario occurs, the farrier should remove the shoe and examine the spot where the nail entered the foot. If a nail enters dermal tissue (even if removed), it causes trauma to the dermal tissue and can seed the area with organisms, which may lead to abscess formation. If the nail has entered the foot inside the sole-wall junction, the owner/trainer should be alerted about the potential problems and the horse could be placed on an oral broad-spectrum antibiotic for 3 to 5 days as a prophylactic measure. Lastly, we have the condition described as a close nail whereby the nail is placed such that it lies against the border of the dermal corium just inside the hoof wall. Pressure against the corium combined with constant movement of the nail against the corium as the horse bears weight may cause an inflammatory response and allow any bacteria that were introduced with the nail to form an abscess as described earlier. There is a lag period of 7 to 14 days or even longer before clinical symptoms or discomfort is observed following the placement of a close nail. Again, treatment would be to establish and promote drainage.

PENETRATING INJURIES TO THE FOOT

Wounds to the solar surface of the foot most often occur when the horse steps on a sharp object, such as a nail. Puncture wounds have been classified according to the depth of penetration (superficial and deep) and the location on the foot.[3–6] Superficial wounds penetrate only the cornified tissue, whereas deep wounds penetrate the germinal epithelium. However, wounds to the sole need only penetrate 1 cm or less to invade germinal epithelium, whereas wounds of the frog may need only 1.5 cm to invade vital structures. Fortunately, the most common wound is a superficial wound of the solar surface of the foot. Deep wounds are more serious and are separated into 3 types based on location. Type I wounds penetrate the sole and may damage P3, whereas type II wounds penetrate the frog and heel area. Type II wounds may involve the deep digital flexor tendon (DDFT), distal sesamoidean impar ligament, navicular bursa (NB), distal interphalangeal joint (DIPJ), the digital flexor tendon sheath (DFTS), and the digital cushion. Type III injuries penetrate the coronary band and may cause septic osteitis of P3, septic chondritis of the collateral cartilages of P3, or septic arthritis of DIPJ. Deep wounds have an increased risk for serious consequences; therefore, the need for early identification of structural involvement and the institution of aggressive medical treatment and early surgical intervention cannot be overemphasized.

CLINICAL PRESENTATION AND DIAGNOSIS

Puncture wounds frequently create marked lameness. The degree of lameness may vary considerably depending on the depth, location, and duration of the wound. Superficial wounds may initially have minimal lameness but can progresses to severe lameness within several days with the development of an infection. In general, puncture wounds that invade the corium become quite painful soon after the injury. Progression to severe non–weight-bearing lameness can occur as the rigid hoof capsule restricts the swelling associated with the inflammatory response. Wounds that involve deeper vital structures, such as P3, or any of the synovial structures, such as the NB, DIPJ, DFTS, or the DDFT, are often rapidly symptomatic. Depth of penetration can be difficult to ascertain when the wound progressives past the horny sole and the severity of the clinical signs do little to help define which structures are involved. Recognizing when the wound occurred and where the wound is located can assist the clinician to choose the most appropriate diagnostic and treatment strategy.

Many horses with puncture wounds to the foot show severe lameness on the affected limb. Increased digital pulses are common; in some cases, the digital pulse may be increased only on the affected side (often with a recent wound). Increased heat may be palpable at the coronary band or over the hoof capsule in the affected limb. Longstanding wounds may lead to a diffuse swelling in the soft tissue of the pastern and above. Early hoof tester application after the injury may reveal focal sensitivity; but over time, a painful reaction may be elicited over the sole region. A visual inspection of the foot will often reveal the source of the lameness. The examination should begin by cleaning the solar surface of the foot. If the offending object, such as a nail, is present, an attempt to obtain a set of radiographs is essential because this can allow the clinician to measure the direction and depth of penetration and evaluate which structures may be involved (**Fig. 4**). Paring the sole with a hoof knife or rasping the hoof wall may reveal the site of the puncture wound or a black tract or crack in the solar surface. Once the surface of the foot is cleaned and the wound or tract is identified, a sterile prep of the foot with an antiseptic detergent and alcohol rinse should be performed. This practice will allow further exploration of the wound, reducing the risk of contaminating the surrounding normal tissue. Probing the wound with a blunt sterile probe or teat cannula can help determine the depth and direction of the wound tract. Radiographs taken with the probe or cannula in place can accurately assess the depth and direction of the wound and possibly the structures affected. If a crack or black tract is found, exploration may lead to an abscess cavity and subsequent drainage. A small-looped hoof knife or a bone curette (# 2) is useful to explore these areas. Locating the entry site of a wound to the frog may prove more difficult because of the elastic tissue of the frog. If a wound is not apparent, hoof testers should be applied in a methodical manner to find a focal point of sensitivity suggestive of the

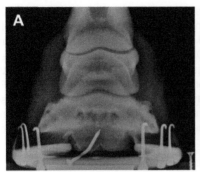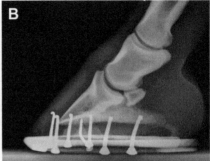

Fig. 4. (*A, B*) If the offending object, such as a nail, is present, an attempt to obtain a set of radiographs is essential because this can allow the clinician to measure the direction and depth of penetration and evaluate which structures may be involved.

puncture site. Removal of as much necrotic tissue and foreign material as possible is important and will dictate the depth and width of the dissection. Visual inspection of the tract is enhanced with the application of a tourniquet to minimize bleeding.

Radiographic examination is indicated with all puncture wounds to identify the presence of concurrent bony involvement, such as fractures, osteitis, and potential sequestrum formation. Gas shadows, debris, and radio-opaque foreign bodies may be seen and indicate the depth and direction of the puncture. More advanced radiographic diagnostic techniques, such as contrast fistulography or contrast arthrography, may be necessary to evaluate a poorly defined wound and to assess the specific structures (especially synovial) that may be involved.

The use of diagnostic ultrasound can be helpful to assess wounds to the foot but is limited to windows provided by the skin at the coronary and the softer tissue of the frog. Given this limitation, diagnostic ultrasound is useful to identify tendon damage and synovial distention and assess the character of the synovial fluid of the DIPJ, NB, and the DFTS. An increase in cellularity and fibrin content in the synovial fluid increases its echogenicity. The presence of gas shadows suggests either an open or breached joint capsule or the presence of gas-producing organisms in the joint fluid. In addition, shadowing artifacts may be visible ultrasonographically, which is suggestive of foreign material, such as wood splinters, or gas commonly seen in coronary band wounds.

Clinical pathologic evaluation of the synovial fluid of the NB, DIPJ, or DFTS is desirable if synovial sepsis is suspected because this will greatly influence the prognosis; however, if the synovial structure is connected to a draining wound, synovial fluid is seldom obtained. With the needle in position in the DIPJ, the joint is injected with a sterile, balanced electrolyte solution in a volume significant to increase fluid pressure within the joint. If fluid is visualized escaping from the wound, it is strongly suggestive that the integrity of the synovial capsule has been compromised and should be considered contaminated and potentially septic. Early diagnosis and aggressive treatment is critical to effectively treat wounds that invade the NB, DIPJ, DFTS, and the DDFT.

Penetrating objects are commonly contaminated with dirt, rust, and manure and this material may be driven deep into the wound. The superficial aspect of the wound frequently seals quickly, especially if the overlying tissue is elastic. Without adequate drainage, an anaerobic environment develops and can promote the growth of anaerobic bacteria. Abscess formation is common, very painful, and requires drainage.

Contamination with the organism *Clostridium tetani* is of particular concern because of the potential threat of tetanus. This disease is difficult to treat successfully, and a history of appropriate vaccination is important. Adequate protection can be achieved by a previous vaccination with tetanus toxoid; however, a booster of toxoid should be given in the event of a puncture wound to the foot. Unvaccinated horses should receive both a tetanus toxoid and a tetanus antitoxin immediately following a puncture wound.

Superficial wounds carry a good prognosis and can have dramatic resolution of lameness within 24 to 48 hours following drainage, whereas deeper wounds require surgical debridement. Superficial wounds and infections are effectively treated by establishing drainage, soaking the foot in an Epsom salt solution, poulticing the foot until drainage has ceased, and protecting the foot until the hoof capsule defect has healed. Farriers are often asked to treat puncture wounds to the solar surface of the foot. Because of the serious complications that can occur following puncture wounds, it is this authors' opinion that when dermal tissue is involved and requires debridement, a veterinarian should become involved in the case. Any delay in the initiation of the appropriate treatment can have serious consequences. Debridement may be painful and necessitates the use of local analgesia at the level of the palmar digital or abaxial sesamoid nerves. In addition, the procedure may cause hemorrhage, which can be minimized when a tourniquet is applied. Regional perfusions are becoming more frequently used to increase the concentration of antibiotics in the foot and require veterinary involvement. Medications, such as antibiotics and antiinflammatory drugs, may be indicated and will need a veterinarian's prescription. If a farrier were to treat an established infection in the hoof, it would be perceived as practicing veterinary medicine and the farrier could be held liable. Farriers are often asked to place a shoe with a removable treatment plate on the foot with a puncture wound for protection but at the same time allowing access for daily treatment. As drainage ceases and the puncture wound begins to cornify, the farrier will be asked to place a pad between the hoof and shoe for protection until healing is complete.

SEPTIC PEDAL OSTEITIS AND SEQUESTRUM FORMATION

Puncture wounds to the sole of the foot can introduce bacteria and debris to the solar surface of P3 and frequently produce a fracture or a septic pedal osteitis. Septic pedal osteitis involves bone lysis of P3 and accompanied by the presence of purulent exudate (which differentiates this condition from nonseptic pedal osteitis).[7] The presence of traumatized periosteum in conjunction with bacterial contamination and poor vascularity of fracture fragments results in an increased incidence of sequestrum formation and osteitis in P3.

The clinical examination may reveal a draining tract that leads to P3. Occasionally, a horse that is on systemic antibiotics and antiinflammatory medications will not manifest significant lameness and drainage until the medications are discontinued. Radiographs will demonstrate the affected area and reveal the presence of an osteitis or sequestrum (**Fig. 5**). If necessary, a fistulogram can be performed to evaluate the tract for a foreign body or to assess the amount of undermined sole.

Surgical drainage and debridement of the infected bone and necrotic soft tissue is necessary for the wound to heal. Wounds to the sole can be safely explored and debrided with the horse standing using local analgesia. The horse should be placed on systemic antibiotics and antiinflammatory medication before surgery. The surgical approach should follow the draining tract and allow adequate exposure for removal of the sequestra and to establish ventral drainage. If there is no visible draining tract,

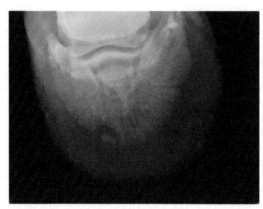

Fig. 5. Radiographs will demonstrate the affected area and reveal the presence of an osteitis or sequestrum.

a radiograph with radio-opaque markers can be placed on the sole and a radiograph taken to map out the approach to the affected bone. An area of sole 1 to 2 cm in diameter should be removed around the puncture site in a conical fashion so that the tract can be completely explored unless radiographs suggest the osteitis/sequestrum is larger. Regional perfusion with broad-spectrum bacteriocidal intravenous antibiotics can also be performed after tourniquet placement and before beginning surgery. Abnormal, discolored bone should be removed by curettage. A culture of the infected bone should determine the appropriate antibiotic therapy, although a mixed growth of several bacterial species can be expected from a contaminated wound. The removal of all infected/affected material is important for the resolution of the drainage and appropriate wound healing. Removal is usually directed by site and by the feel of the bone when debrided with a curette. A tourniquet placed at the fetlock and proximal sesamoid bones should be used to minimize bleeding and allow the surgeon to better distinguish between normal and abnormal tissue. Daily inspection of the surgery site is helpful to determine if further debridement of abnormal discolored tissue or bone is necessary. Daily, or every other day, bandage changes are necessary to protect the wound from trauma/desiccation, to apply pressure to the wound surface minimizing excessive granulation tissue formation, to absorb exudate, and to maintain dressings/topical medication on the wound surface. Heavily contaminated wounds and larger wounds often need frequent dressing changes. Some horses remain uncomfortable after surgery and require stabilization of the hoof capsule and removal of the affected sole from direct weight bearing. However, bandaging alone does little to provide stability to the hoof capsule. The application of a roll of 2 to 3 in casting tape around the perimeter of the hoof wall at the ground surface or the placement of a therapeutic shoe can provide additional stability to the hoof capsule. Most often, a straight bar shoe with quarter clips will suffice and may include a treatment plate. Alternatively, a heart bar shoe (with a treatment plate) may be used to allow some weight bearing to be transferred from the hoof wall to the frog. These shoes should be applied such that access to the wound is maintained.

Maggot debridement is a nontraumatic, minimally invasive, optional method that has been described in the literature. It can be used after sharp debridement to assist with the removal of necrotic tissue from a deep extensive foot infection. This therapy should be used in conjunction with and after surgical debridement. Maggot therapy may decrease healing time in postsurgical P3 debridement.[8]

The prognosis for soundness depends on the cause of the infection, its duration, and the adequacy of surgical debridement. In one report that evaluated septic osteomyelitis of the distal phalanx it was found that up to 25% of the distal phalanx can be removed and the horse has the potential to be sound.[9]

PENETRATING INJURIES TO THE NAVICULAR AREA

Penetrating injuries to the frog can extend to the DDFT and, depending on the direction, can extend into the NB, DIPJ, or DFTS. These injuries are considered potentially career ending and even life threatening because potential sepsis within any of these synovial structures carries a guarded to poor prognosis. Sepsis of any synovial structure requires immediate and aggressive treatment. Wounds to this area have the potential to involve synovial structures, therefore, careful evaluation for synovial involvement is warranted. If a radio-opaque foreign body, such as a nail, is still in place, survey radiographs should be considered essential to determine the depth and direction of the penetration and the structures involved. The survey radiographs should include a 0° dorsopalmar, lateromedial, 60° dorsopalmar (navicular and P3 technique), and palmaroproximal palmarodistal (skyline) views. At least 2 radiographs taken in orthogonal planes with the probe or foreign object in place are necessary to define the correct depth and direction of the penetration. If the object has been removed before the examination, then careful scrutiny of the foot may reveal the puncture site. A sterile metal probe can be used to evaluate the course and extent of the wound (**Fig. 6**). Contrast fistulography and contrast arthrography/bursagraphy are radiographic techniques that can be used to further define the wound and any involvement with the DDF and the synovial structures. Contrast fistulography is useful to assess the depth and direction of the tract by placing a catheter into the wound and injecting contrast material under pressure. The path the contrast travels typically follows the path of the puncture wound. Contrast arthrography/bursagraphy is performed by injecting contrast material into the DIPJ, NB, or DFTS independently to demonstrate synovial membrane integrity. If the wound has breached one of these synovial structures, the contrast material may leak from the synovial space into the subcutaneous tissues and into the tract (**Fig. 7**).

Diagnostic ultrasound can be useful in assessing wounds that involve the frog. A careful evaluation with a high-frequency microconvex or linear probe placed on a carefully pared frog may demonstrate gas shadows present in the soft tissues of the foot, in

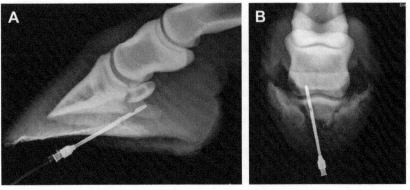

Fig. 6. (*A, B*) A sterile metal probe can be used to evaluate the course and extent of the wound.

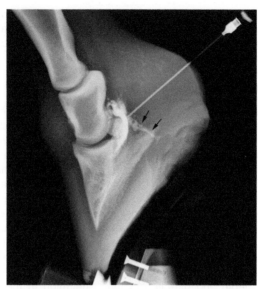

Fig. 7. Contrast arthrography/bursagraphy is performed by injecting contrast material into the DIPJ, NB, or DFTS independently to demonstrate synovial membrane integrity. The black arrows demonstrate contrast leakage into a penetrating injury that entered the navicular bursa.

the navicular bursa, or DIP joint and should be considered confirmation of penetration and probable contamination. Diagnostic ultrasound can also be used in conjunction with a probe or needle placement because metal content from each creates a shadowing artifact that can be visualized and followed in real time to determine the involvement of key structures. In addition, sequential ultrasonographic examinations may be used to assess the response to therapy as evidenced by changes seen in the character and quantity of the synovial fluid. When surgically placing a closed-suction drain to the distal extent of the sheath, it may be assisted by the use of ultrasound. This practice is particularly important to evaluate the effectiveness of a closed-suction apparatus in collecting the accumulating fluid formed within the DFTS.

The aseptic collection of a joint-fluid sample at a site remote from the wound is recommended in all cases if possible. An increase in total cell count (>30,000–40, 000 cells/ μL) with a predominance of neutrophils and an elevated total protein concentration (≥3 g/dL) are good indicators of sepsis. Gram staining of the joint fluid may demonstrate free bacteria in the joint fluid. The fluid should be submitted for bacterial culture and antibiotic sensitivity testing. Samples of synovial fluid from the coffin joint, digital flexor tendon sheath, and navicular bursa should be obtained. Even if one or more of these structures is contaminated, the prognosis is improved by early diagnosis and immediate and aggressive medical and surgical therapy.

Medical therapy includes broad-spectrum systemic antibiotics, nonsteroidal antiinflammatories, and should include appropriate surgical debridement (both endoscopically and the wound), copious lavage of the synovial structure, regional perfusion of antibiotics, and intraarticular antimicrobial medication.

The diagnostic findings dictate which surgical procedure is performed. With wounds involving the frog that are not thought to involve a synovial structure, the cornified tissue overlying the puncture site should be removed and the tract explored to its limit.

A probe or the careful injection of new methylene blue dye into the tract can be used to guide dissection. Wounds thought to involve any of the synovial structures of the foot should be approached endoscopically for debridement and lavage. This procedure must be performed under general anesthesia. At the same time, regional perfusion with an appropriate antibiotic can be performed. Endoscopic examination of the synovial structures have been described in detail elsewhere.[10] In addition to endoscopic debridement and lavage, the site of the wound is debrided by sharp dissection and all devitalized tissue is resected. After completion of the procedure, an antibiotic is injected into the affected synovial structure.

Historically, infections of the navicular bursa have been managed by a procedure termed a street nail surgery. This procedure involves creating a funnel or square-shaped window in the frog with layer-by-layer dissection through the digital cushion to expose the DDFT. In this process, all devitalized tissue around the puncture wound is debrided (**Fig. 8**). If the puncture wound seems to continue through the DDFT, then a longitudinal incision that separates the tendon fibers is made in the DDFT to allow exposure to the navicular bursa. Any portion of the tendon that seems necrotic or devitalized is resected. The navicular bursa is opened and lavaged. Careful placement of the window through the DDFT over the flexor cortex of the navicular bone is critical to avoid entering the coffin joint distal to the navicular bone (through the impar ligament) and the palmar/plantar pouch of the coffin joint or the digital flexor tendon sheath proximal to the navicular bone. The flexor tendon sheath and coffin joint should be distended to determine if there has been inadvertent penetration of either structure.

Postoperative care is a critical aspect of the street nail procedure. Lavage of the bursa/joint/sheath and both regional perfusion and intraarticular/intrathecal antibiotics should be performed at the clinician's discretion (the authors use a course of once-daily perfusions for 3 days and then every other day for 3 days continuing until clinical improvement is seen). The surgical wounds and the dissected frog wound should be maintained under a sterile bandage and changed daily until the discharge begins to diminish. Convalescence after the street nail procedure is much longer than for horses treated using endoscopic lavage of the navicular bursa. The street nail wound will take substantially longer to fill in and will require much more frequent and intense postoperative care. Those horses that require a street nail procedure may have a cancellous

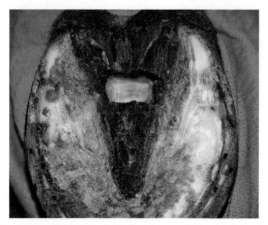

Fig. 8. Street nail surgery. This procedure involves creating a funnel or square-shaped window in the frog with layer-by-layer dissection, through the digital cushion to expose the DDFT. In this process, all devitalized tissue around the puncture wound is debrided.

bone graft harvested from the tuber coxae and packed into the wound attempting to promote the obliteration of dead space, prevent ascending contamination, and provide a scaffolding into which cells can migrate during wound healing.[11]

Horses with involvement of the DDFT often require some form of heel elevation following surgery to reduce the strain placed on the tendon. Reducing the strain in the DDFT is important because it seems to allow the horse to be more comfortable. In the short term, elevating the heels may be accomplished by placing the foot in a commercial wedge shoe with a cuff (Nanric, Inc, Versailles, KY, USA), taping multiple (3–4) 3° pads together, and then attaching them to the bottom of the bandage or having the farrier build a heel elevation shoe with a removable treatment plate (**Fig. 9**). Every attempt to provide comfort on the affected foot should be undertaken to reduce the likelihood of mechanical (overload) laminitis from developing in the contralateral limb. Eventually, a therapeutic shoe can be applied that incorporates this heel elevation (multiple 3° wedge pads) and a treatment plate to expedite wound dressing changes. Box stall rest is recommended for at least 60 to 90 days. Loading the DDFT may take the form of hand walking but is dictated by the comfort level of the horse and the degree of tendon involvement seen at surgery. The shoe is reset every 2 weeks, with removal of one pad depending on the comfort level of the horse at each shoeing. This progressive removal of the wedges should produce a gradual elongation of the DDFT muscle tendon unit and remodeling of the scar that forms in the wound to improve the deformability of the tendon and scar tissue.

When financial constraints limit more involved therapy, transcutaneous lavage of the navicular bursa, with ingress/egress of fluid and antibiotic via an 18-gauge, 3.5-in spinal needle can be attempted often in combination with regional perfusion (**Fig. 10**). However, it is important to impress on the client that this procedure is likely to be effective only in early cases with minimal contamination and, even then, the success rate is much lower than for surgical exploration and lavage.

In an early report, horses with NB sepsis treated with appropriate surgical debridement within 4 days after injury had a reasonably good prognosis. A recent article has reported good success with arthroscopic exploration of the NB in lieu of the more aggressive street nail procedure.[12–14] Cases involving a hind limb are more likely to

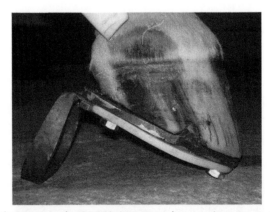

Fig. 9. Reducing the strain in the DDFT is important because it seems to allow the horse to be more comfortable. In the short term, elevating the heels may be accomplished by placing the foot in a commercial wedge shoe with a cuff, taping multiple (3–4) 3° pads together, and then attaching them to the bottom of the bandage or having the farrier build a heel elevation shoe with a removable treatment plate.

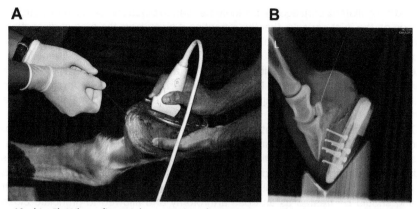

Fig. 10. (*A, B*) When financial constraints limit more involved therapy, transcutaneous lavage of the navicular bursa, with ingress/egress of fluid and antibiotic via an 18-gauge, 3.5-in spinal needle, can be attempted in conjunction with regional perfusions. Confirmation of placement of the needle into the navicular bursa with radiographic or sonographic control is critical.

return to previous activities than those involving a forelimb. When the DDFT and related structures are involved, the prognosis is more guarded. The most common and serious mistake made in the management of these cases is the initial use of a conservative approach.

INFECTION OF THE COLLATERAL CARTILAGES (QUITTOR)

Lacerations, puncture wounds, abscesses, and occasionally hoof wall cracks can involve the collateral cartilages of the foot. Wounds that involve the collateral cartilage may cause cartilage necrosis, which leads to chronic infection of the cartilage. Trauma to the lateral cartilage above the coronet, such as the horse stepping on that area, may also lead to necrosis of the lateral cartilage. Infection of the collateral cartilages of the foot is termed quittor and seems to be most common in draft breeds but can occur in any breed. A chronic nonhealing wound or abscessation located above the coronary band over the lateral cartilage with intermittent purulent discharge is the usual clinical presentation. The diagnosis is based on the location, clinical signs of swelling, and drainage from the affected cartilage. The primary differential diagnosis is chronic foot abscess. However, the drainage site for quittor is usually *above* the coronary band, whereas most submural abscesses (gravel) drain from the coronary band. The drainage will generally have a putrid odor. Lameness can be severe, especially when pressure increases from the accumulation of purulent material within the infected structures. But as with foot abscesses, once drainage occurs, the lameness seems to diminish.

The collateral cartilages have a poor blood supply, so healing of these tissues is slow. Furthermore, because much of the cartilage lies within the hoof capsule, it is difficult to establish effective drainage, making quittor a surgical disease. The treatment of choice is surgical excision of all infected tissue and the establishment of adequate ventral drainage in conjunction with broad-spectrum antimicrobials. The wound should be cultured but it is likely to grow a mixed population of bacteria. The surgeon can culture the infected cartilage when removed at surgery, which will give a more accurate culture and sensitivity.

A proximally based, curved incision is made to access the infected cartilage. Meticulous dissection is necessary because the palmar pouch of the DIPJ is located just axial to the collateral cartilages. It is recommended to place the foot in traction to place tension on the joint capsule, thereby retracting it away from the area of dissection.[11] Surgical dissection can also be assisted by carefully injecting new methylene blue into the draining tract to clearly identify the affected tissue. Complete removal of all diseased cartilage may necessitate removal of a portion of the proximal hoof wall, which can be performed with a Dremel tool (robert Bosch Tool Corporation, Racine, WI, USA) or trephine, while taking care to preserve the germinal tissue of the coronary band.

Once the dissection is complete, the DIPJ should be distended with sterile balanced electrolyte solution and the wound assessed for fluid leakage that would indicate the loss of integrity in the joint capsule. If the DIPJ capsule is breached, then the prognosis is diminished and the joint should be treated as if contaminated. If the joint capsule can be closed, then an attempt should be made to do so. If closure is not possible, the wound should be treated as an open arthrotomy and allowed to granulate closed. The skin incision is closed primarily, if possible, and drainage portal is established ventrally through the hoof wall if necessary.

The prognosis is guarded because it can be difficult to remove all of the infected tissue. The incision is at risk of dehiscence, which can complicate those cases when the coffin joint was invaded. If the coffin joint is invaded, then treatment becomes much more aggressive and must address the principles previously discussed.

The second author (S.E.O.) has taken a different approach on a limited number of cases. The foot is anesthetized on the affected side using an abaxial nerve block. A hole is drilled through the outer hoof wall distally extending into the dermal tissue directly below the wound. A long hemostat is used to thread a thin Penrose drain from the wound through the dermal tissue exiting through the opening created in the distal outer hoof wall. The following day, the wound is flushed with sterile saline and sterile maggots are introduced into the wound at the coronet, dry gauze pads are placed over the wound, and the foot is bandaged. The bandage is changed every second day to remove exudate, and the maggots are changed at weekly intervals. Therapy is continued until the wound becomes dry and closes.

INTRAVENOUS REGIONAL PERFUSION FOR SEPTIC PROCESSES IN THE DIGIT

Infection can be a serious complication in wounds involving the foot. Foot infections can be difficult to treat because they often are polymicrobial, the organisms may be resistant to multiple commonly used antibiotics, and the infected area may be poorly vascularized (owing to its inherent structure or because swelling of the infected soft tissues within the rigid hoof capsule impedes vascular flow). Infection is enhanced in the presence of damaged devitalized tissue, hematoma formation, avascular bone, or foreign material (including soil and fecal matter).

Sepsis, vascular compromise, and a drop in pH as a consequence of inflammation and ischemia may prevent adequate delivery or activity of antibiotics in the infected tissue. Furthermore, vascular compromise increases the risk of sequestrum formation, which can promote bacterial proliferation.

Intravenous regional perfusion (IVRP) involves the delivery of an antibiotic to a selected region of the limb via the venous system. The infused volume is delivered under pressure to ensure the distribution of the fluid to all vascular spaces in the region distal to the tourniquet. Retention of the antibiotic in the venous space for 20 to 30 minutes allows diffusion into surrounding tissues than may otherwise have inadequate blood flow. During IVRP of the distal limb, it is possible to achieve antibiotic concentrations in the tissues that are 25 to 50 times the minimum inhibitory concentration required to kill most pathogenic bacteria.[15] Thus, with this technique, it is possible to achieve therapeutic concentrations of antibiotic even in necrotic tissue.

TECHNIQUE

Regional perfusion of the digit can be performed in the standing horse (**Fig. 11**).[15,16] The skin over the medial or lateral digital vein is aseptically prepared. A local anesthetic can be use to create a local skin block where the catheter is to be placed. A catheter is aseptically placed in the digital vein; most clinicians use a 20-gauge catheter, placed in the lateral digital vein. A tourniquet or Esmarch bandage is applied at the fetlock. An extension set is attached to the catheter and infusion is begun. Ideally, the antibiotic chosen is determined by culture and sensitivity results. Frequently, however, the results are not available when the first perfusion is performed. The clinician must, therefore, rely on clinical judgment and select an appropriate antibiotic based on the most likely organisms involved. The antibiotics most commonly used for IVRP include amikacin (0.5–1.0 g), gentamicin (1 g), potassium penicillin (10 million units), Timentin (1 g), and cefazolin (1–2 g). Whichever antibiotic is selected, the amount to be delivered (eg, 1 g amikacin) is diluted in 20 to 30 mL of sterile balanced electrolyte solution. The antibiotic solution is infused over 30 to 60 seconds, but the tourniquet is left in place for a total of 20 to 30 minutes before it is removed.

IVRP can be performed as a single treatment or repeated as often as necessary until clinical improvement is seen or the patency of the digital veins becomes compromised. The most common complication with IVRP is injury to the vasculature and soft tissues either from catheterization or perivascular leakage of the solution and subsequent local reaction.

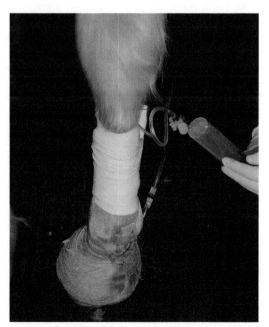

Fig. 11. A catheter is aseptically placed in the digital vein; most clinicians use a 20-gauge catheter, placed in the lateral digital vein. A tourniquet or Esmarch bandage is applied at the fetlock.

INTRAOSSEOUS INFUSION

Intraosseous regional perfusion is an alternative to IVRP. It has the advantage of avoiding the repeated use of regional vessels. This technique does not achieve as high a tissue level of antibiotic concentration as regional perfusions, although it is still significantly higher than the minimum inhibitory concentration. There is the added risk of a fracture through the drill hole. With this technique, the antibiotic solution is infused into the intraosseous space. After aseptic skin preparation, local anesthesia, and a stab incision through the skin and periosteum, a 4-mm diameter hole is drilled through the cortex of the bone adjacent to the septic process. An intraosseous infusion needle or the male adaptor of an intravenous extension set is wedged into the hole and the antibiotic solution is infused into the medullary cavity. Unfortunately, the bones of the digit exist within or close to the hoof capsule, which makes easy access to the surface of the bone for the placement of the drill hole difficult.

REFERENCES

1. Parks AH. Form and function of the equine foot. In: O'Grady SE, editor. The veterinary clinics of North America, vol. 19. Philadelphia: W.B. Saunders Co; 2003. p. 285–307.
2. O'Grady SE. Strategies for shoeing the horse with palmar foot pain. In: Proceedings 52nd Annu Conv Am Assoc of Equine Pract 2006. p. 209–12.
3. Richardson GL, Pascoe LR, Meagher D. Puncture wounds of the foot in horses: diagnosis & treatment. Comp Cont Educ Pract Vet 1986;8:S379–87.
4. Stashak TS. Adams' lameness in horses. 4th edition. Philadelphia: Lea and Febiger; 1987. p. 703–10.
5. Redding WR. Pathological conditions involving the internal structures of the foot. Equine Podiatry. St. Louis (MO): Saunders/Elsevier; 2007.
6. Boado A, Kristoffersen M, Dyson S, et al. Use of nuclear scintigraphy and magnetic resonance imaging to diagnose chronic penetrating wounds in the equine foot. Eq Vet Educ 2005;17(2):62–8.
7. Moyer W, O'Brien TR, Walker M. Non-septic pedal osteitis—a cause of lameness and a diagnosis. In: Proceedings 45th AEEP 1999;45. p. 178–9.
8. Morrison SE. How to use maggot debridement therapy for infections in the horse. In: Proceedings 51st AEEP 2005. p. 51.
9. Gaughn EM, Rendano VT, Ducharme NG. Surgical treatment of septic pedal osteitis in horses: nine cases (1980-1987). J Am Vet Med Assoc 1989;195:1131–5.
10. Cruz AM, Pharr JW, Bailey JV, et al. Podotrochlear bursa endoscopy in the horse: a cadaver study. Vet Surg 2001;30:539–45.
11. Honnas CM, Welch RD, Ford TS, et al. Septic arthritis of the distal interphalangeal joint in 12 horses. Vet Surg 1992;21:261–8.
12. Wright IM, Smith MR, Humphrey TC, et al. Endoscopic surgery in the treatment of contaminated and infected synovial cavities. Equine Vet J 2003;35:613–9.
13. Schneider RK, Bramlage LR, Mecklenburg LM, et al. Open drainage, intra-articular and systemic antibiotics in the treatment of septic arthritis/tenosynovitis in horse. Equine Vet J 1992;24:443–9.
14. Schneider RK, Bramlage LR, Mecklenburg LM, et al. Retrospective study of 192 horses affected with septic arthritis/tenosynovitis. Equine Vet J 1992;24:436–42.
15. Whitehair KJ, Blevins WE, Fessler JF, et al. Regional perfusion of the equine carpus for antibiotic delivery. Vet Surg 1992;21:279–85.
16. Palmer SE, Hogan PM. How to perform regional limb perfusion in the standing horse. In: Proceedings 45th AAEP 1999;45. p. 124–7.

Treating Laminitis
Beyond the Mechanics of Trimming and Shoeing

William R. Baker Jr, DVM

KEYWORDS

- Laminitis • Horse shoeing • Trimming • Farriery

KEY POINTS

- Laminitis is typically classified into developmental or prodromal, acute, subacute, and chronic phases.
- Scientific evidence regarding the pathophysiology of laminitis does exist, but it is often conflicting and dependent on the clinician's interpretation/understanding of the study or the model used for inducing laminitis.
- The diagnosis of laminitis consists of obtaining an accurate history, performing a thorough physical examination, and taking good-quality radiographs.
- The use of radiographs for diagnosis and interpretation of laminitis is an absolute necessity for the clinician.
- Laminitis is one disease that requires the assembly of a team consisting of the veterinarian, the farrier, and the owner to be successfully treated.

Laminitis has now obtained the auspicious state of being classified as the most debilitating disease that affects the equine species. This title is certainly well earned, if not overdue, in recognition of the devastation this disease produces. Laminitis is approaching the number one reason for euthanasia, a close second to colic in the horse. With these facts in mind, it is surprising that laminitis research lags behind many other disease processes in the horse. Since there are many different causes of laminitis, it is difficult to reproduce a research model in a laboratory setting that is all encompassing. Perhaps one reason for the lack of solid scientific evidence concerning laminitis is that it is generally a sequelae to a preexisting disease process, though it may occur as a primary disease. It may be helpful for the clinician to examine the current knowledge and perceptions of laminitis in the horse. By examining current theories and perceptions about laminitis, the clinician should be able to form a more logical approach to diagnosis and treatment. This article will present an overview of the current ideas regarding the pathophysiology, diagnosis, and treatment of laminitis

The author has nothing to disclose.
Equine Associates LLC, 693 Unadilla Highway, Hawkinsville, GA 31036-0810, USA
E-mail address: wrbaker@comsouth.net

Vet Clin Equine 28 (2012) 441–455
http://dx.doi.org/10.1016/j.cveq.2012.05.004
0749-0739/12/$ – see front matter

in a manner such that it pertains to the clinician-making decisions on a routine basis, much as occurs in the author's practice, and the importance of establishing communications between the veterinarian, farrier, and horse owner.

PATHOPHYSIOLOGY

Current perceptions and knowledge of laminitis as a disease state often depend on the clinician's personal perspective. Scientific evidence regarding the pathophysiology of laminitis does exist, but it is often conflicting and dependent on the clinician's interpretation/understanding of the study or the model used for inducing laminitis. Three common research models known to induce laminitis are black walnut heartwood extract (BWHE), oligofructose, and insulin.[1–3] Each of these models differs in the pathophysiology proposed for initiating a laminitis response. BWHE, which is the oldest model, uses endotoxemia and a vascular pathophysiology theory to explain the onset of laminitis.[4] The oligofructose model studied by Van Epps and Pollit involves an enzymatic pathway in which methyl-metalloproteinases cause separation of the epithelial cells from the basement membrane, which may subsequently lead to mechanical collapse of the lamellae.[2] The insulin model relies on endocrine pathology and the failure of normal homeostatic mechanisms of insulin production and the ability of cells to respond to insulin.[3] A more recent theory proposed involves the systemic inflammatory response syndrome.[5] This syndrome proposes a pathogenesis for lamellar destruction based on the pathogenesis of organ failure as noted in human sepsis.[5]

The vascular model proposed by Hood and the enzymatic model proposed by Pollit are those most widely accepted among clinicians.[4,5] These models have merit and research data to support them; however, neither can fully explain the pathophysiology across the spectrum of causes for laminitis nor has a trigger factor that would initiate the process been discovered. The insulin model is very specific as to the cause and effect of insulin variations in the horse and its relationship to laminitis; therefore, it is difficult to reconcile with the understanding of the pathophysiology of laminitis that has arisen from the carbohydrate and black walnut models of the disease. The systemic inflammatory response syndrome explains the pathophysiology across numerous instigating causes but needs further research to verify its existence in the horse. One author has listed 80 causes, predispositions, and pathways of laminitis.[6] The list, although not definitive, certainly alludes to the difficult task of assigning one pathophysiology for laminitis that would be all encompassing. Indeed, it is likely that there is more than path of entry into the disease process. Also of importance is whether there is a final common pathway through which the different initiating factors come together; a common pathway would have significant implications for medical management of the disease in the future.

DIAGNOSIS AND CLASSIFICATION

Historically, laminitis has been described as a problem in the horse as far back as 350 BC.[7] It has been given many different names over the course of history but the symptomatology has allowed us to classify all of these diseases as one we currently refer to as laminitis. Diagnosis of the disease has not significantly changed in centuries. The horse with laminitis has the classic stilted gait, reluctance to move, bounding digital pulses, excessive heat associated with the hooves and coronary band, and obvious weight-bearing pain.[8–10] What has changed over the centuries is our ability to recognize the symptoms earlier and to classify different stages and severities of the disease along with our clinical expectations of response to therapy.

The diagnosis of laminitis consists of obtaining an accurate history, performing a thorough physical examination, and taking good-quality radiographs. A complete blood cell count, serum chemistry, and specific endocrine assays may also be helpful in specific cases; however, the history and physical examination should be used to determine their necessity.

History

The history should determine whether this is an initial episode, a recurrence, or an exacerbation of a continuing episode. It should also include any preexisting conditions the horse may have, such as a retained placenta, a recent colic episode, or a recent change in exercise routine. The environment should be taken into account as well as the season of the year. For example, it has been shown that fructan levels, which are implicated as an instigating factor in certain types of laminitis, in the grass change from season to season and during periods of draft or heavy rainfall.[11] Attempting to obtain an etiology from the history is always worthwhile by asking questions such as: What are the current feeding routines of the horse and has anything changed? Have any medications or vaccinations recently been given to the horse? Is the horse on any long-term medications? Has the horse been diagnosed with any disease processes? Has there been a history of trauma recently or in the past associated with the laminitis? Has the horse had excessive stress or been shipped a long distance? These types of questions can give an insight into the cause of the laminitis and how to initiate treatment. Taking a good history is often overlooked by the clinician eager to treat the horse but well worth the time as valuable information can be obtained.

Physical Examination

The physical examination is performed with both the eyes and the hands of the clinician. Observing the horse's stance and willingness to move can give information as to the degree of pain the horse is experiencing.[12] Observing the horse's body and head position when the clinician is lifting a limb from the ground gives clues as to the degree of discomfort. Palpation for increased heat in the foot and at the coronary band as well as an increase in the digital pulse characteristics give the clinician an idea of the intensity of the inflammation occurring.[8] Palpation of a depression immediately proximal to the coronary band in the distal pastern can give the clinician an indication of the possibility of distal displacement. The prudent and artful use of hoof testers can also give the clinician valuable information. Hoof testers provide the clinician with insight to the areas of the sole that are most painful. In the laminitic horse, the toe and quarters are typically the most sensitive, but this can vary depending on the severity and type of laminitic episode. The appropriate use of hoof testers on the horse is an acquired skill and is dependent on the competency the clinician has for using the tool; therefore, the information obtained should be interpreted with the skill level the clinician has with hoof testers.

Radiology

The use of radiographs for diagnosis and interpretation of laminitis is an absolute necessity for the clinician. It has become the standard in the diagnosis and care of the laminitic horse. Diagnosis and treatment of laminitis without radiographs, in this author's opinion, are extremely difficult. Proper radiographic technique and positioning are essential to obtain a diagnostic image.[13] The 2 essential views for laminitis are the lateral and the dorsopalmar or dorsoplantar. The shoes of the horse do not have to be removed to obtain diagnostic radiographs. The lateral views should be taken with both feet on blocks of equal height and the focal beam directed through the solar margin of the distal phalanx (DP). A zero film distance should be obtained when taking this view to avoid magnification. Any variation from this technique will result in unnecessary artifacts and false information.[13]

The Dorso-Palmar (Plantar) view should also be taken with the feet on blocks with the focal beam centered on the solar (distal) border of the DP. Once again, there should be a zero film to subject distance to prevent magnification and artifact development. There are some excellent publications on proper radiographic technique of the equine foot, which the author highly recommends.[14] The foot should have appropriate markers along the dorsal wall of the hoof and at the apex of the frog. Many types of radiopaque markers have been used; however, the author recommends the use of barium paste for this purpose. These markers are essential in obtaining the necessary measurements for evaluating laminitis. The markers allow a definitive determination of the outer hoof wall and the relationship of the apex of the frog to the apex of the DP. The measurements used to evaluate the laminitic patient are the coronary/extensor distance (CE), the sole depth at both the dorsal solar margin of the DP, and the palmar solar margin of the DP, sole depth (SD), the horn/lamellar distance (H/L zone, the thickness of the hoof capsule plus underlying dermis and subcutaneous tissue), and the palmar angle of the DP (PA, also referred to as the angle of the solar margin of the DP) (**Fig. 1**).[15]

The classic dorsal angle measurement, in this author's opinion, is not as important as it was once considered and may serve to cause confusion and misinformation about the condition of the foot. The classic method of measuring the dorsal angle of the DP as the only determinate of displacement and severity of the disease does not take into account many important parameters. The SD, the CE and the H/L zone must all be accounted for to accurately portray the severity of the laminitic episode. The dorsal angle can be influenced by the deformation of the outer hoof wall and gives no useful information to the clinician or farrier when mechanically altering the position of the DP with the ground surface. The CE, SD, H/L zone, and PA allow radiographs to be standardized and allow communication between clinicians to be more productive. Horses with distal displacement will show an increase in the CE, a decrease in SD, and an increase in the H/L zone (**Fig. 2**). Phalangeal rotation will show an increase in the H/L zone and a decrease in SD at the apex of the DP and an increase in the PA in the palmar aspect of the DP (**Fig. 3**). These measurements allow the clinician to communicate treatment alternatives and prognosis more effectively to both the farrier and the owner. Radiographs are not only useful for diagnosis but also may help with prognosis and guidelines for an appropriate treatment plan.

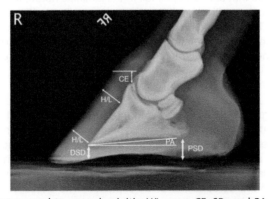

Fig. 1. The parameters used to assess laminitis: H/L zone, CE, SD, and PA.

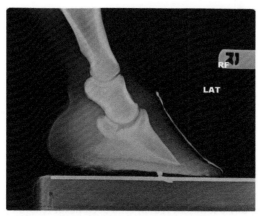

Fig. 2. An example of distal displacement, sinking. The CE measurement has increased, and the SD at the dorsal margin of the DP has decreased.

The recent advances in venography have allowed a more accurate diagnosis, classification, and prognosis in conjunction with plain radiographs.[16,17] Venography has been alluded to being therapeutic in some cases, but this has not been observed by the author.[17] The author uses venography extensively with laminitis cases with its principal value being prognosis. The venogram allows the visualization of the vascular perfusion of the digit and a method of monitoring progress over 3- to 7-day time spans. Radiographs typically take weeks to months to demonstrate progression of a given case. Venography thus allows a significant advantage as to changing treatments, implementing new treatments, and upgrading the prognosis of the patient (**Figs. 4** and **5**).[18]

CLASSIFICATION OF THE LAMINITIC PHASES

Laminitis is typically classified into developmental or prodromal, acute, subacute, and chronic phases.[4] The chronic phase can further be classified into compensated and noncompensated subcategories.[19] These classifications do not necessarily change

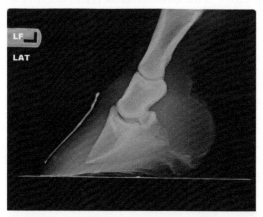

Fig. 3. Phalangeal and capsular rotation demonstrating an increase in the H/L zone, more so distally than proximally, and a decrease in SD at the dorsal margin of the DP.

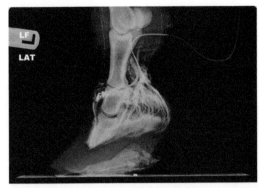

Fig. 4. Venogram of the left fore; note the apex of the DP below the circumflex vessels. In the author's opinion, this is sufficient reason for a deep flexor tenotomy. Also note the lack of visualization of the capillary complex ventral to the apex of the DP and the effusion along the dorsal surface.

the way a diagnosis of laminitis is derived but provide for institution of more specific treatments and a prognosis of the individual case. The understanding of the basics for these classifications gives the veterinarian a starting point for which treatment decisions and prognosis can be made and a beginning by which the farrier and the owner can become involved. With an accurate classification, the farrier understands his or her role in therapy and the owner understands the prognosis and expectations toward resolution of the case.

Developmental Phase

The developmental phase is the period between the initiating insult and the onset of acute lameness that is diagnosed as laminitis.[4] The length of time of this phase can range from 24 to 60 hours with the average range of 40 hours.[13] It is during this time that the triggers or mechanisms that lead to laminitis become active. The importance of the developmental phase lies in the ability of the clinician to intervene before the laminitic mechanisms become active. Pollit has shown that intervention at this phase, experimentally, can prevent laminitis from developing or decrease its severity.[11,20] The problem is the developmental phase is asymptomatic. As a result,

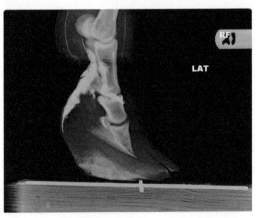

Fig. 5. Example of a failed venogram due to failure of the catheter to remain in the vein.

the clinician rarely has the opportunity to institute therapy at this stage. The developmental phase is usually associated with circumstances or conditions that predispose the horse to laminitis.

Examples of these conditions would be colitis, retained placenta, heat exhaustion, carbohydrate overload, metabolic disease, pituitary tumors, and toxic plant ingestion. The veterinarian must rely heavily on the knowledge of predisposition of laminitis from the presenting complaint. Carbohydrate overload is the easiest to recognize because owners have been educated as to the tendency of this syndrome to cause laminitis; however, it is still very dependent on owner knowledge, recognition of the incident, and willingness to treat aggressively and quickly. The reluctance to treat these horses quickly is likely a result of the absence of clinical signs and also because a number of cases that have received no treatment do not develop laminitis.

Acute Phase

The acute stage of laminitis has been very well defined as to duration and symptomatology.[4,8,21] In the acute phase, the first signs of discomfort are noticed. The shifting of weight by the horse, the classic stilted gait, or the reluctance to move is noted. The classic clinical observations include increased pulse rate and intensity of the palmar digital vessels, an increase in temperature around the coronary band, and hoof tester sensitivity over the toe and quarter area. The acute phase has a time duration of 24 to 72 hours, which has been observed consistently and is deemed definitive of this phase.[4] This is the phase in which enough cellular damage can occur to result in displacement of the DP. If displacement has not occurred in 72 hours, the horse moves into the subacute phase and the prognosis improves; however, if displacement occurs during this phase, the prognosis is dramatically altered.

Subacute Phase

The subacute phase occurs after 72 hours have elapsed with no displacement of the DP.[4] This phase can last days to months. In the subacute phase, repair of the damaged lamella tissue begins. Depending on the severity of laminar damage, the subacute horse can either return to previous levels of performance or progress to a chronic stage. The horse in the subacute phase that has severe lamellar destruction can continue a slow ongoing degeneration to the point of digital collapse, the destruction of the lamellar bond, and subsequent displacement of the DP. Laminitis resulting from metabolic disease, steroid induced displacement, and supporting limb laminitis is more likely to be associated with a more insidious degeneration of the lamellae. The average duration of the subacute phase has been quoted as 8 to 12 weeks.[4] The author finds this time period to be optimistic. During this phase, the lamellar attachment is tenuous; therefore, it is possible for the horse to suffer structural failure due to a weakened lamellar interface. In the subacute phase, the goal is to promote stabilization of the digital structures and to alleviate pain through the use of support to the foot. This can be accomplished by several techniques ranging from Styrofoam pads or wooden shoes to the classic heart bar shoes. The author typically will not shoe horses with a subacute case and will rely on a pad made from dental impression material (Advanced Cushion Support; Nanric, Lawerenceburg, KY, USA) taped to the bottom of the foot. If the horse continues to improve through the subacute phase, the prognosis for return to the previous level of work improves dramatically.

Chronic Phase

The chronic phase of laminitis occurs when there is sufficient structural damage within the hoof capsule to cause digital collapse.[4] This phase is certainly the most complex and has the worst prognosis of the 3 phases. The laminitic horse can progress to the chronic phase from the acute phase or the subacute phase. It is not uncommon for a laminitic horse to progress from the acute to the chronic phase within 24 hours of onset of the symptoms.[4] Any displacement, rotation, or sinking should be considered to place the horse in the chronic phase and be treated appropriately.[22] The chronic phase is frequently severe because the disease at this stage is multifaceted. The vasculature of the foot is now compromised along with significant tissue degeneration. The tendinous attachment of the DP begins to exert deleterious forces within the hoof capsule, creating more damage. The necrosis occurring from tissue destruction increases and sepsis is always a significant possibility. The severe pain associated with this stage of the disease makes it very difficult to treat. The variation of clinical and radiographic findings within the chronic phase has led to the creation of 2 subcategories: chronic compensated and chronic noncompensated. Chronic compensated laminitis can be defined as a condition in which significant and permanent laminar damage has occurred and there is displacement of the DP, but the foot has become stabilized.[19] Morrison defined "stabilized" in chronic laminitis as the DP no longer displacing and the foot generating new sole and wall tissue.[23] Although the hoof growth can be distorted, the horse is usually "pasture sound" due to the DP being stable within the hoof capsule. In the chronic noncompensated laminitic horse the DP continues to move, causing shearing and compression to the lamellar and vascular tissue.[19] This compression on the sole and coronary band can result in abscesses or sepsis of the foot. These cases are usually in severe pain. All these diagnostic classifications are used to establish a treatment protocol, to provide the owner with information about the current status of the horse, and to establish a prognosis for quality of life and future athletic ability.

TREATMENT
Acute Laminitis

Therapy of the laminitic horse should be based on the diagnostic classification of the patient. Therapy for acute laminitis is designed to alleviate the pathophysiologic events that are occurring. Most therapies are designed to mitigate endotoxemia and the systemic inflammatory response syndrome and to improve circulation and alleviate pain. These mechanisms are interrelated and the alleviation of one can lead to the alleviation of another. For instance, the use of nonsteroidal anti-inflammatory drugs not only alleviates pain but also exerts an antiendotoxic effect by blocking systemic and local inflammation.[24] Acepromazine is the only vasodilator proved to be effective in the increase in digital blood flow of the horse; however, it has only been proved to increase digital blood flow in healthy horses and not specifically in horses with laminitis.[25] Pharmacologic uses of drugs such as dimethylsulfoxide as an anti-inflammatory agent and oxygen radical scavengers have had clinical success. The use of cryotherapy has recently gained favor; however, cryotherapy has only been shown to ameliorate experimentally induced laminitis and only in the developmental stage.[26] In the acute phase, there are no published data showing the benefits of cryotherapy, only anecdotal evidence. If cryotherapy is to be instituted as therapy in the acute phase, it needs to be continuous distal limb cryotherapy for up to 7 days.[26] Although there may be some benefits to cryotherapy such as analgesia and reduction of inflammation and enzymatic activity, the author has found the correct use of this therapy to be very difficult in the field. There is a wide array of drugs that have been used successfully and unsuccessfully to treat acute laminitis in the horse. When confronted with a disease with a poorly understood pathophysiology, the tendency is to resort to anecdotal therapies.

The other component of treating the acutely laminitic horse is mechanical support. The principal objectives of mechanical support are to provide axial support to unload the diseased lamellar tissue, to reduce the distracting forces on the laminar interface, and to reduce the forces on the foot applied by the deep flexor tendon.[20] The foot must be supported in an effort to stabilize the structural components of the foot. This is usually accomplished by stall rest and pads of some description. Pads routinely used are Styrofoam, gauze, Lilly pads, or those made with a synthetic polymer. There is a commercial wedged cuffed shoe available that can be used in acute cases (Redden Ultimate; Nanric Inc, Versailles, KY, USA). Other methods used to support the foot include the use of wooden shoes, foot casts, glue-on shoes, and heart bar shoes. Appropriate trimming of the foot before application of any of the above-mentioned techniques can aid in the reduction of damaging mechanical forces. Beveling of the toe to reduce stresses on the dorsal hoof wall is a common technique. The heels may be elevated to reduce stresses from the deep digital flexor tendon and shift weight bearing to the quarter and heels.[27] The elevation relaxes or disengages the forces applied to the DP by the deep digital flexor tendon helping to prevent further separation of the lamellar tissue. If sufficient elevation cannot be achieved or dorsal rotation is severe enough, a deep digital flexor tenotomy should be considered to alleviate the tensional forces applied to the DP. The goals with both the pharmacologic and supportive techniques in the acute stage of laminitis are to alleviate pain and prevent further tissue destruction, provide stabilization of the digit, and promote an optimal healing environment.

Subacute Laminitis

The objectives of treatment in the subacute phase of laminitis are continuation of support for stabilization, promotion of a proper healing environment, and prevention of reoccurrence of the inflammatory process. These objectives are achieved by continuing to monitor the horse's condition with serial radiographs, adjusting the support technique and trimming as needed, and providing appropriate pharmacologic treatment and rest. While in the subacute phase, the horse has a higher probability of recovery to soundness; however, there is also a very real chance that, if not properly supported and treated, the horse can suffer digital collapse with devastating consequences. Continued monitoring and treatment are absolutely critical in the subacute stage of this disease. Concurrent systemic diseases also need to be addressed during this stage to prevent a recurrence of the inflammatory process or a slow deterioration of the lamellar tissue causing digital collapse. In the horse with a supporting limb laminitis, the clinician must continue to address the contralateral limb in an effort to prevent continuing laminar degeneration. In the horse with metabolic syndrome, changing the diet, monitoring endocrine levels such as insulin, Adrenocorticotrophic hormone (ATCH), and cortisol, and using appropriate medications are needed to prevent recurrence.

Chronic Laminitis

Chronic laminitis may be classified as any damage to the digit that is sufficient enough to cause digital collapse and repositioning of the DP.[28] Digital collapse may occur in the acute or subacute stages and has no definitive time line. A horse may go from the acute stage to the chronic stage in 24 hours or it may be months into the subacute stage when changes occur to cause digital collapse. The chronic phase of laminitis can be divided into 2 subcategories, compensated and noncompensated, due to the varying degrees of supporting structural damage and the variation of displacement of the DP. Displacement of the DP can take the form of dorsal capsular rotation, distal displacement, or mediolateral rotation.[29] All 3 forms can occur in any combination and are directly dependent on the severity and location of supporting structure damage that has occurred. The occurrences of varied manifestations of chronic laminitis have lead to many different treatment protocols. The central theme with all these techniques is alleviation of pain and comfort of the horse. When a horse has progressed into the chronic stage of laminitis, the probability of return to athletic performance is questionable. Treating the horse with displacement has 2 objectives. The first is realignment of the DP with the hoof capsule. The second is to provide stabilization of the supporting structures and the DP and thus comfort to the horse. These 2 are not mutually exclusive and often one will follow the other.

The first step in treatment is to determine the type and severity of structural damage and displacement. The most important determinant in the long-term outcome is the degree of instability between the DP and the hoof wall.[28] Radiographs and venograms help to provide this information. Radiographs and venograms provide information as to the position of the DP within the hoof capsule, remodeling of the DP, and indications of digital sepsis formation. The venograms provide information as to vascular integrity, vascular flow, and the creation of lamellar wedging. When all data from the physical examination, radiographs, venograms, and any laboratory profiles have been obtained, then an informed decision can be made whether to treat the chronic laminitic horse or whether humane destruction should be considered. If treatment is undertaken, the first step should be realignment of the DP. This involves trimming to realign the solar surface of the DP with the ground surface of the hoof capsule (**Figs. 6** and **7**). The objective of the trim is to also alleviate stresses to the most damaged portion of the foot, usually the dorsal hoof wall, by transference of weight to the less affected area of the hoof capsule. Trimming is also used to aid in reestablishment of the vascular flow within the digit by alleviation of compression of the circumflex vasculature by the dorsal border of the DP. These principles are useful for dorsal capsular phalangeal rotation but are not for the horse with distal displacement (sinkers). Horses that have undergone distal displacement have a total loss of structural support within the hoof capsule. This author has no knowledge of a trim technique to aid these cases. The objectives of trimming for a chronic laminitic horse with capsular rotation are to reduce the load on the most severely affected area of the foot, transfer weight bearing to the least severely affected area of the foot, increase breakover, and realign the solar surface of the DP with the ground surface of the hoof capsule.[29]

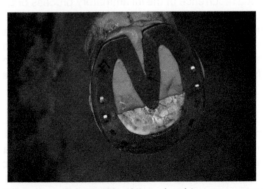

Fig. 6. Application of a heart bar shoe with advanced cushion support to prevent necrosis of the frog.

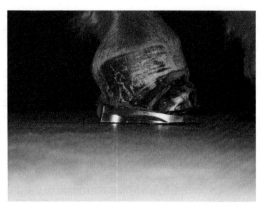

Fig. 7. De-rotation and application of the 4-point rail shoe in a horse with chronic laminitis with severe dorsal rotation.

After the appropriate trim is applied, the foot is ready to be shod. Therapeutic shoeing is once again most helpful for the chronic laminitic foot with dorsal phalangeal rotation and has had limited success in horses with mediolateral rotation of the DP. Therapeutic shoeing of the horse with distal displacement, in this author's opinion, is not beneficial. The principles applied to therapeutic shoeing of the chronic laminitic horse are moving the point of breakover palmarly, to provide support for the entire ground surface of the foot, and elevation of the heels (see **Fig. 7**; **Fig. 8**). Moving the breakover palmarly decreases the stresses on the dorsal lamellae during movement and shifts the weight bearing to the caudal portion of the foot. Supporting the entire ground surface of the foot is done in an attempt to shift the weight-bearing distribution across the total surface and thereby unload the stress on the hoof wall. Elevation of the heels decreases the tensional forces applied by the deep flexor tendon and decreases the stresses on the dorsal lamellae. The types of shoes used to accomplish these objectives are many and varied. The heart bar shoe has been referenced in literature as early as 1894 and is still used today.[30] The egg-bar shoe, D-bar shoe, EDSS (Equine Digit Support System Inc, Penrose, CO, USA) shoe, 4-point rail shoe, wide web aluminum shoe, wooden shoe, reverse shoe, and the composite shoe have all been used for the treatment of chronic laminitis. All of these shoes have had their

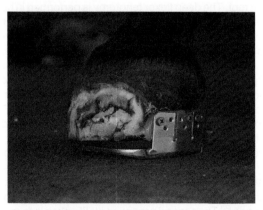

Fig. 8. Application of a natural balance shoe (Equine Digit Support System Inc, Penrose, CO, USA) post hoof wall resection. Laminitis with rotation secondary to white line disease.

successes and their failures. This can be attributed to the complexity of the chronic laminitic foot and the comfort the farrier has with the shoe used. All of these shoes incorporate the 3 principles previously mentioned; however, some have more merit with certain principles than others.

For example, the heart bar shoe has more emphasis on total support of the ground surface of the foot and little on heel elevation. The wooden shoe incorporates all 3 principles: breakover, ground support, and heel elevation. Modification to all of these shoes has occurred over time to incorporate all 3 principles with varying degrees of success. A pad placed on the palmar surface of the foot is a common adjunct to the shoe. A moldable pad system that will fill all parts of the sole, frog, and bars is the most beneficial in this author's opinion. The moldable pad such as a synthetic polymer, impression material (Advanced Cushion Support, Nanric), or a polyurethane (Equipak, Solpak; Vettec, Oxnard, CA, USA) literally molds to the ground surface of the foot, providing even weight distribution.

These materials can also be molded to provide elevation where needed, such as in the heel, or they can be used inside a foot cast. Elevation of the heels has been used to aid in the comfort of the horse during realignment of the DP. Providing elevation to the heels is thought to reduce the stresses on the dorsal lamellae caused by tension applied to the DP from the deep digital flexor tendon. The degree of elevation varies from case to case and is a matter of preference of the clinician to a large extent. The range of elevation commonly used by this author is 3° to 12°. The choice of shoes is determined by the severity of the case and the degree of past success the veterinarian or farrier has had with the shoe. As mentioned before, it is very seldom a shoe will be used without modification and additions so as to be most appropriate for the case at hand and applying the therapeutic principles of chronic laminitis. The author has used the 4-point rail shoe with impression material (Advanced Cushion Support; Nanric Inc, Versailles, KY, USA), the EDSS, natural balance shoe (Gene Ovincek, Penrose, CO, USA), the wooden shoe, and the heart bar shoe to treat specific chronic laminitic cases (see **Figs. 6–8**).

The shoe chosen for each case and the modifications made, such as changing breakover and providing medial to lateral breakover, are dependent on the information gathered during the history, physical examination, and radiographs. A realignment shoeing technique using glue-on shoes and impression material has been described for use in severe cases.[18] Surgeries such as the deep flexor tenotomy, transfixation casts with hoof wall ablation, and resections are also used to alleviate the stresses and mechanical forces applied to the foot. The deep flexor tenotomy is performed in horses with phalangeal rotation. Indications for this procedure include continuation of rotation of the DP despite conservative therapy, penetration of the solar surface by the DP, or a void of contrast media on the dorsal surface of the DP on a venogram.[18] The transfixation cast with hoof wall ablation is usually reserved for the most severe distal displacement cases. This technique involves complete removal of the hoof wall followed by placing 2 stainless steel Steinman pins at oblique angles in the metacarpal or metatarsal bone. A cast then incorporates the foot and the pins, forming a half-limb cast. This reestablishes blood flow to the foot by removing all restrictions of the hoof wall and redistributes the weight of the limb to the metacarpus or metatarsus via the pins and cast.

The practice of resection of the dorsal wall was proposed by Chapman and Platt[9] to alleviate pressure from serous fluid accumulation following lamellar separation. More recently, it has been proposed that the purpose of strategic wall resection is to alleviate the compromise displacement of the DP causes to the circulation of the coronary, lamellar, and solar coria.[23] The second proposed justification is to prevent the coronary corium from becoming necrotic, causing horn growth to become permanently damaged. The use of selective hoof wall resection has shown to improve circulation and hoof wall growth.[16] The use of foot casts in the horse with chronic laminitis may be beneficial if the horse has poor hoof wall quality.[31–33] A foot cast can supply ground surface support and stabilization when a shoe cannot be attached. The use of glue-on shoe techniques are often used with many of the above-mentioned shoes as a modification for an individual case with poor hoof wall quality or a problem with nailing the shoe. There can be some repair of the laminar structures when placed in the appropriate environment; however, in the severe cases the vascular alteration of the digital circulation is such that a complete recovery is unlikely. The alteration of vascular flow within the foot can lead to chronic abscesses, sepsis and altered hoof wall growth. The author has used most of the techniques mentioned with varying degrees of success and finds the determining factors for a successful outcome to be the degree of severity, the appropriateness of the technique, and the expectations of the owner.

VETERINARIAN-FARRIER-OWNER RELATIONSHIP

Laminitis is one disease that requires the assembly of a team to be successfully treated. This team consists of the veterinarian, the farrier, and the owner. This trio creates a very diverse group and presents challenges in communication and the approach to treatment of the laminitic horse. The veterinarian approaches laminitis from a systemic disease and physiologic point of view. The farrier typically approaches laminitis from a mechanical viewpoint, taking into account the physics applied to the horse's foot. The owner approaches laminitis from an emotional attachment to the horse and information obtained from veterinarians, farriers, nutritionists, friends, trainers, as well as other sources. With the Internet age, the availability of a diverse range of opinions on laminitis and the treatment of laminitis has become one click away. It is easy to understand how confusing the situation can become when placed under the stress of caring for a horse with laminitis; therefore, it is critical that the veterinarian present the diagnosis, treatment plan, and prognosis in an easy-to-understand format. The veterinarian must be able to translate into everyday language the progression of the disease, how it is affecting the horse, how can it be treated, and what are the expectations for the quality of life.

The veterinarian's relationship with the owner is important. The veterinarian should be honest and direct with his or her opinions and prognosis. This is usually a very difficult time for the owner and he or she will have a host of questions. The veterinarian should try to answer all the owner's questions and make him or her feel a part of the team process. The owner always has the last decision as to caring and treatment and it is up to the veterinarian to make sure the owner has the best possible information available to make that decision. Before treatment is initiated, the owner needs to understand the severity, the prognosis, and the estimated costs. The veterinarian, as the team leader, needs to communicate these facts clearly and needs to inform the owner that at anytime the horse's condition might change. It is the veterinarian's responsibility to provide all the details available and projected costs and possible outcome of the case.

When treatment is initiated, the veterinarian then needs to establish a rapport with the farrier and make sure the treatment plan is understood. Farriers should be chosen not only for their experience but also for their willingness to work with the veterinarian as a team and openness to new ideas. Treatment of laminitis is not a standardized cookbook technique. Treatment often involves changing, adjusting, and being creative. The farrier can bring fresh ideas and insights to the team. The farrier's role may be limited in the acute case that responds, but in the chronic case the farrier may be involved with the horse for years. The farrier and the veterinarian should approach these cases with optimism. As treatment progresses, the veterinarian needs to communicate frequently with the owner and the farrier, updating condition, prognosis, and further treatment recommendations. The cost of treatment needs to be updated as well.

SUMMARY

Laminitis is a disease that has been afflicting horses throughout recorded history. There is still much that is not known concerning the mechanisms that actually initiate a laminitic episode and there is no one proven treatment protocol. However, more is understood now compared with 10 years ago in regard to pathophysiology and causative agents of laminitis, and research continues. Several research models have been developed that reliably induce laminitis; however, none encompass all the inciting causes, predispositions, and pathways of laminitis. The ability to use modern technology has allowed clinicians to more accurately assess the severity of damage that has occurred, allowing more appropriate classification of the disease phase. The appropriate classification of the laminitic phases has produced more appropriate treatment protocols and, to some extent, a more accurate prognosis.

Current research has focused on prevention and the developmental phase of laminitis. There have been advancements in treatment in the acute phase. New analgesics have been introduced and cryotherapy has been proposed as a possible treatment for the acutely laminitic horse. The chronic phase has seen advances with current shoeing techniques, and advances in product technology have made horses more comfortable and made small strides in rehabilitation. The irreparable damage that is often seen in the chronic laminitic horse makes significant therapeutic advances difficult, but perhaps not impossible with further technology progress. It is hoped that one day the mechanisms or inciting factors of laminitis will be discovered and prevented.

The importance of veterinarian, farrier, and owner communication cannot be overstated. With all the available information at our fingertips, it is a necessity to establish clear and open communications to avoid confusion as to treatment and prognosis. Veterinarians need to work with the highly trained farrier and well-informed owner and incorporate them into a working team, using their skills and abilities.

REFERENCES

1. Galey FD, Whiteley HE, Goetz GE, et al. Black walnut toxicosis: a model for equine laminitis. J Comp Pathol 1991;104(3):313–26.
2. Van Eps AW, Pollitt CC. Equine laminitis induce with oligofructose. Equine Vet J 2006;38(3):203–9.
3. Asplin KE, Sillence MN, Pollitt CC, et al. Induction of laminitis by prolonged hyperinsulinaemia in clinically normal ponies. Vet J 2007;174(3):530–5.
4. Hood DM. The pathophysiology of developmental and acute laminitis. Vet Clin North Am Equine Pract 1999;15(2):321–43.
5. Eades SC. Overview of current laminitis research. Vet Clin North Am Equine Pract 2010;26(1):51–63.
6. Heymering HW. 80 Causes, predispositions, and pathways of laminitis. Vet Clin North Am Equine Pract 2010;26:13–9.
7. Dunlop RH, Williams DJ. Veterinary medicine: an illustrated history. St Louis (MO): Mosby; 1996.
8. Baxter GM. Laminitis. In: Robinson NE, editor. Current therapy in equine medicine. 3rd edition. Philadelphia: WB Saunders; 1992. p. 154–60.
9. Chapman B, Platt GW. Laminitis in the horse. In the Proceedings of the American Association of Equine Practitioners 30th Annual Meeting, Dallas (TX); 1984. p. 99–105.

10. Swanson TD. Clinical presentation, diagnosis, and prognosis of acute laminitis. Vet Clin North Am Equine Pract 1999;15(2):311–9.
11. Geor RJ. Current concepts on the pathophysiology of pasture-associated laminitis. Vet Clin North Am Equine Pract 2010;26(2):265–78.
12. Obel N. Studies on the histopathology of acute laminitis. Thesis. Uppsala (Sweden): Almqvist & Wiksells Boktryckeri AB; 1948.
13. Redden RF. Radiographic imaging of the equine foot. Vet Clin North Am Equine Pract 2003;19:379–92.
14. Redden RF. Equine podiatry: monograph series, radiography of the equine foot. Versailles (KY): Nanric; 2002.
15. Rucker A. The digital venogram. In: Floyd AD, Mansmann RA, editors. Equine podiatry. St Louis (MO): Saunders; 2007. p. 328–46.
16. Rucker A. Equine venography and its clinical application in North America. Vet Clin North Am Equine Pract 2010;26(1):167–77.
17. Redden RF. Possible therapeutic value of digital venography in two laminitic horses. Equine Vet Educ 2001;13:125–7.
18. D'Arpe L, Bernardini D. Digital venography in horses and it clinical application in Europe. Vet Clin North Am Equine Pract 2010;26(2):339–59.
19. Herthel D, Hood DM. Clinical presentation, diagnosis, and prognosis of chronic laminitis. Vet Clin North Am Equine Pract 1999;15(2):376.
20. Reilly PT, Dean EK, Orsini JA. First aid for the laminitic foot: therapeutic and mechanical support. Vet Clin North Am Equine Pract 2010;26(2):451–8.
21. Colles CM, Jeffcoat LB. Laminitis in the horse. Vet Rec 1977;100:262.
22. Parks A, O'Grady SE. Chronic laminitis: current treatment strategies. Vet Clin North Am Equine Pract 2003;19:393–416.
23. Morrison S. Chronic laminitis foot management. Vet Clin North Am Equine Pract 2010;26(2):425–46.
24. Belknap JK. The pharmacologic basis for the treatment of developmental and acute laminitis. Vet Clin North Am Equine Pract 2010;26(1):116–24.
25. Leise BS, Fuger LA, Stokes AM, et al. Effects of intramuscular administration of acepromazine on palmar digital blood flow, palmar digital arterial pressure, transverse facial arterial pressure, and packed cell volume in clinically healthy, conscious horses. Vet Surg 2007;36:717–23.
26. Van Eps A. Therapeutic hypothermia (cryotherapy) to prevent and treat acute laminitis. Vet Clin North Am Equine Pract 2010;26(1):125–33.
27. Parks A, Balch OK, Collier MA. Treatment of acute laminitis, supportive therapy. Vet Clin North Am Equine Pract 1999;15:363–74.
28. Hunt RJ, Wharton RE. Clinical presentation, diagnosis, and prognosis of chronic laminitis in North America. Vet Clin North Am Equine Pract 2010;26(1):141–53.
29. O'Grady SE. Farriery for chronic laminitis. Vet Clin North Am Equine Pract 2010; 26(2):407–23.
30. Dollar JAW. Shoeing after laminitis. A handbook of horseshoeing. New York: William R Jenkins; 1898. p. 352.
31. Hunt RJ. Equine laminitis: practical clinical considerations. In: Proceedings. Am Assoc Equine Pract. San Diego (CA). 2008;54:347–53.
32. Hunt RJ, Brandon CL, McCann ME. Effects of acetylpromazine, xylazine, and vertical load on digital arterial blood-flow in horses. Am J Vet Res 1994;55:375–8.
33. Pollit CC, Pass MA, Pollitt S. Batimastat (BB-94) inhibits matrix metalloproteinases of equine laminitis. Equine Vet J 1998;26:119–24.

Index

Note: Page numbers of article titles are in **boldface** type.

Vet Clin Equine 28 (2012) 457–466
http://dx.doi.org/10.1016/S0749-0739(12)00074-0
0749-0739/12/$ – see front matter © 2012 Elsevier Inc. All rights reserved.

vetequine.theclinics.com